Pasteur, Microbes, Vaccines, the Truth

ANDRÉ HUAN

Published by ANDRÉ HUAN, 2021.

PASTEUR, MICROBES, VACCINES, THE TRUTH

First edition. January 29, 2021.

ISBN: 979-8223369714

Written by ANDRÉ HUAN.

Dear reader,

This book aims to shed light on the indoctrination, that most health professionals have been victims of for more than 140 years, since a chemist named Louis Pasteur, instigated his false and deadly theory of vaccination.

This theory, which is based on four dogmas whose falsity has been demonstrated, has in fact led modern medicine down a dangerous path that removes responsibility from the human beings that we are, claiming to protect them when it can kill them, either radically (sudden infant death syndrome), or slowly (cancers of all kinds).

And, if we compare the planet to the human body, **the vaccine cancer of France** has sent its metastases to every other country on Earth.

Certainly, some tribes in the depths of the Amazon have yet to escape the evil syringe, but the World Health Organization is saddened by this and is implementing programs that will ensure that no one escapes.

And if human beings are finally beginning to realize the poisoning they are inflicting on their planet, due in part to the billions of tons of pesticides that have been dumped over the past 60 years, they have not yet realized that they are experiencing the same thing in their own bodies. But let's rather say that we prevent him from realizing it by lying to him, by conditioning him, by indoctrinating him.

A journalist said recently about Daesh: ***"In the face of propaganda, you need information."*** The parallel with the vaccination is obvious, in the sense that all those who dare to inform and question the sacrosanct Pasteurian religion are denigrated and ostracized by society.

When it comes to the protection of the Earth, Resistance fighters such as Mr. José Bové are threatened with prison when they oppose, among other things, the introduction of genetically modified organisms into agriculture, but they are not called mad.

It's something else when it comes to Resistance fighters that we are to the introduction of pus (the real name that vaccines should have but which would be much less selling) into our own bodies, we are called irresponsible, obscurantist or sects all by ourselves!

But the latest fashionable maneuver of the proponents of the vaccine doctrine is to rank us among the partisans of the **"conspiracy theory"**! This is the only argument they have left to defend their religious dogmas since they cannot refute the scientific evidence of their falsity. The method has been widely tested; when one cannot oppose arguments, one discredits their authors.

Seed or vaccine merchants, same objective: money, again and again, regardless of the health consequences of the products they sell.

The former have obtained a ban on the sale of seeds they do not produce themselves, the latter the obligation to buy their virus concentrates, no matter if this obligation is in total contradiction with the laws of France!

But as Buddha said to his disciples: **"Do not believe at once what I tell you, check it."** May you examine this book in the light of the truth by checking all the information it contains. The actors of the vaccine religion will never tell you this. To them, the less you know, the better. Keeping people in the dark, is the best way to keep a hold on them. So they hope that their messages will be convincing enough that you won't even think to check their contents.

For its part, if this book helps to prevent even one sudden death of a single infant, one child with autism or one person with multiple sclerosis, it will have achieved its goal.

The fact that you have bought it shows that you are wondering about the effectiveness and especially the safety of vaccinations and that you are more or less escaping the deadly indoctrination that the Pasteurian religion has been undertaking for more than a century and a half on our minds.

"And yet it's spinning! " In the 16th century, there was a strong belief that the Earth was stationary, and that it is at the center of the universe, this theory is the universal rule, and any contrary assertion is condemned, as is the one who utters it.

"And yet it kills! " In the 21st century, it is firmly believed that vaccination is safe, and protects against diseases and epidemics, this theory is the universal rule and any statement to the contrary is condemned, as is the person who utters it.

By his abjuration, Galileo escaped the death penalty, and on June 16, 1633 the verdict was final:

"The said Galileo will be called upon to abjure, condemned to life imprisonment, and summoned to stop discussing his theories under penalty of relapses. His work, like that of Copernicus, will be put on the Index. The sentence will be sent to all members of the clergy and will be read in the presence of as many of those who profess the art of mathematics as possible."

Today, under penalty of 6 months in prison and a fine of 3,750 euros, it is forbidden to refute the vaccine dogma, the fruit of the famous "single thought" that is denounced but shared by almost all the media and all political leaders, whatever their political persuasion.

Galileo knew that resisting the Inquisition was a lost cause. Holding on to his life, he ended up acknowledging his guilt and his "heretical depravity" as the Holy Office put it. Three times he swore he was wrong:

"I do not support and I abandon the opinion of Copernicus; I have no more doubts and I hold that of Ptolemy to be very true. Yes, the Earth is fixed, at the center of the world. And then, I am in your hands, do with me what you please."

Broken, Galileo ended his plea with a humble prayer, begging for clemency and kindness from his judges.

It was not until the years 1820-1830 that the Church definitively and completely accepted the idea that the Earth revolved around the Sun. She rehabilitated Galileo three and a half centuries later, in 1992.

21st century: Since Galileo was the heretic who had to be silenced at all costs, five hundred years later, there are a few million "heretics" on the planet, who claim (for those who can do so without risking their profession), that vaccination is indeed heresy.

The most brilliant swindle, the most successful masquerade, the most subtle manipulation, and above all **the most deadly medical catastrophe of the 20th century,** these are some of the adjectives that can be attached to the vaccination myth, because it is indeed a myth.

In order to preserve their children's health, and avoid ending up in prison for refusing to vaccinate or losing their parental rights, some parents have come to choose to provide them at home with the education, that is denied them by the National Education system. But we still need to have the financial means to be able to do so, **the "freedom" of the French republican motto is not the only one to be flouted, "equality" too!**

LOUIS PASTEUR: THE MEDICAL HERESY

Occasionally, ask your doctor if, during his long studies, he has learned anything about Professor Antoine Béchamp, a contemporary of Louis Pasteur?

Because the whole story of vaccination - starts with these two men. Who were they?

Antoine BÉCHAMP (1818 -1908)

- Pharmacy graduate
- Doctor of Medicine
- Degree in Physical Sciences
- Doctor of Physical Sciences
- Professor of Physics and Toxicology at the École Supérieure de Pharmacie in Strasbourg
- Professor of Medical Chemistry and Pharmacy at the Faculty of Medicine of Montpellier.
- Dean of the Free Faculty of Medicine and Pharmacy of Lille
- Professor of organic chemistry and biological chemistry in Lille

Antoine Béchamp discovered the primordial element and the living cell that he named microzyma. He demonstrated that it could become a bacterium or virus and deduced the bacterial polymorphism. Polymorphism (from the Greek pleon: more abundant, and morphê: form) is the capacity of an organism (essentially bacteria) to take on different forms under certain conditions or under certain influences.

He denounced the error of Pasteur's monomorphism, which led medicine towards a phobia of microbes and neglect of the field.

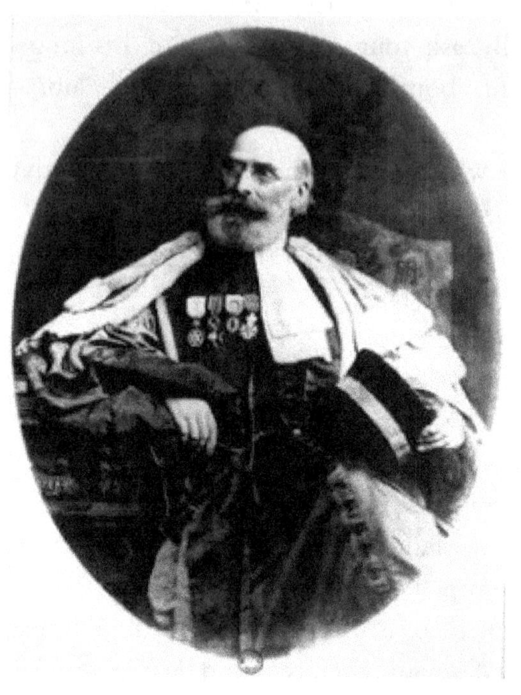

Antoine Béchamp

Louis PASTEUR (1822-1895)

- Doctor of Science

- Aggregate of Physics and Chemistry

An ingenious specialist in public relations and advertising marketing, he appropriated Professor Béchamp's discoveries, by diverting them from their origin. Thus he simply renamed Antoine Béchamp's microzyma into a microbe, claiming to have discovered it!

Then he developed the theory, that the microbe is at the origin of the disease, whereas for Antoine Béchamp and his followers, it is the disease that allows the microbe to express itself.

Pasteur speaks only of "germs" in the air, considers microbes only as agents of disease, and teaches that living organisms are aseptic, readily comparing them to a barrel of wine or beer!

And it is on this total absurdity that all modern medicine is based with the main Pasteurian dogma: one germ = one vaccine!

This is an aberration, because if we prevent a germ from expressing itself spontaneously, it will adapt, transform itself and a new type of disease will appear!

Every year in France, the Telethon collects donations dedicated to research to defeat 5,000 new diseases described as "genetic". How many of these are a direct consequence of mass vaccination campaigns? We will probably find out one day, and that day will open long trials. Because the pirouette of "those responsible but not guilty" cannot continue ad vitam aeternam.

The child did not have rabies!

In elementary school, we were taught that the unfortunate child, had been bitten by a rabid dog and that without the saving bite of Louis Pasteur, he would have inevitably contracted this dreaded disease.

The truth is quite different. Very few people know, that the owner of the biting dog, Max Vone, as well as several other people, who were bitten by this animal on the same day, remained in good health without any treatment, which means in short that the dog was not rabid at all...

The vaccine theory of the whole world is based on this unique and false case!

The height of cynicism, Pasteur passes before the eyes of the members of the Academy of Sciences and the Academy of Medicine, the painting of six children who died of rabies from June 17 to September 24, after having been vaccinated, a painting on which one reads next to the name of each victim, these two poignant words: insufficient treatment...

The total number of deaths from rabies, despite rabies vaccination is, as of November 2, 1886, 53. In France, the average annual number of people who die of rabies before the release of the vaccine is 30.

Pasteur believed in spontaneous generation!

This man, who is still considered today as a savior of humanity, and whose name is glorified by the smallest town in France by giving it to a street, a square, an avenue or a boulevard, this man shared the popular belief of his time, illustrated as follows: *"if you put flour and wet rags in a pot of earth, in a few days a generation of mice, male and female, will come out of it, perfectly constituted."*

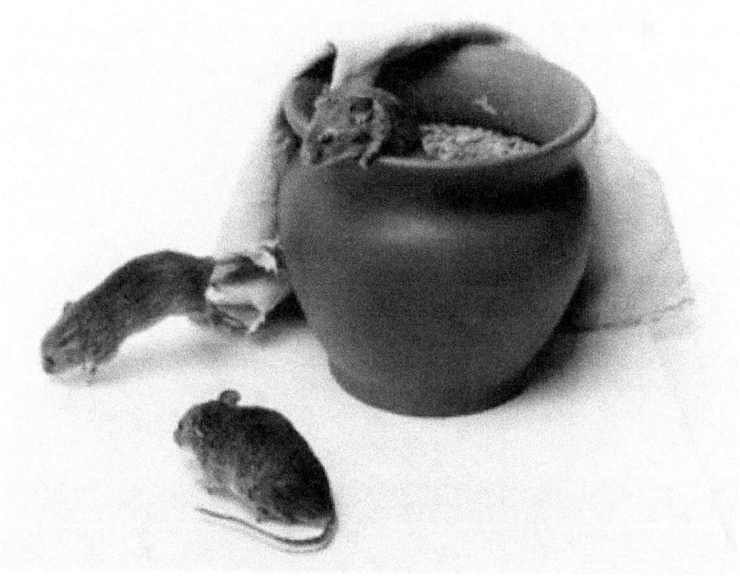

This did not prevent him from writing later, after turning his jacket: *"the spontaneous generation will not recover from the mortal blow I dealt it."*

This says a lot about the "great scientist" quality attributed to the chemist.

Witness, the excerpts from the long letter written by Antoine Béchamp, 84 years old, when Pasteur had been dead for more than four years. He replies to a certain Doctor Vitteaut who, in a press article, thought he was paying tribute to him, by presenting him as Pasteur's precursor.

DES
MICROZYMAS

ET DE LEURS FONCTIONS

AUX DIFFÉRENTS AGES D'UN MÊME ÊTRE

PAR

Joseph BÉCHAMP

DOCTEUR EN MÉDECINE

Professeur à l'École et à Faculté de médecine ; Membre de la Société de médecine et de chirurgie
pratiques ; Membre de la Société médicale d'Émulation.

MONTPELLIER

C. COULET, LIBRAIRE-ÉDITEUR
LIBRAIRE DE LA FACULTÉ DE MÉDECINE
ET DE L'ACADÉMIE DES SCIENCES ET LETTRES
Grand'Rue, 5

PARIS

ADRIEN DELAHAYE, LIBRAIRE-ÉDITEUR
Place de l'École-de-Médecine

1875

Paris, May 190

Mr. Doctor.

I received your "scientific-religious question" *... If I did not hold you in very high esteem, because of your good intentions, I would not write to you. I will do so in all sincerity... to complain, to justify myself, and to disillusion you.*

Let me first tell you that Mr. Denys Cochin misled you about Mr. Pasteur, either through ignorance, or bad faith...

It is obviously to make your hero grow up, and to pay me a compliment, that you made me Pasteur's precursor: I do not know where you took this opinion, that you had already expressed elsewhere, and that I had not taken up; but since you reproduce it, in conditions that I hold offensive, suffer that I tell you this: I am Pasteur's precursor as the stolen one is the precursor of the fortune of the rich, happy and insolent thief, who mocks and slanders him.

Here is to disabuse you: *I pose in fact that Pasteur, whatever you say, according to Mr. Denys Cochin, did not discover, any of the facts of which you glorify him, and that he did not introduce into Science any new truth.*

You could have convinced yourself of this, by reading the preface of the book on Microzymas (1883). A single example is enough to demolish all the scaffolding, built to erect a monument to the glory of the one you call "our Pastor". It is the one that proves, ***that he neither discovered the germs of which you speak,*** *nor solved the ancient question of spontaneous generations.*

If this is true, nothing remains of your assertion, that Pasteur proved that life does not appear without a germ, that in the living world therefore every living being proceeds from a cell, "omnis cellula a cellula".

Well no! Mr. Doctor, this is not true, *and Mr. Denys Cochin, on whose authority you rely, if he said this, has not been a true historian.*

To be convinced of this, one need only look at the Memoir on Lactic Fermentation which he published in 1858. There, you will see that Pasteur stated iteratively that lactic yeast, vibrios and brewer's yeast, which is a true cell, *SPONTANEOUSLY BORN, from the albuminoid matter of the fermentable medium.*

Is this clear? *Thus in 1858, Pasteur, being able to choose between two hypotheses each having adherents: that of germs and that of sponteparity, pronounced himself in favour of spontaneous generation, without even discussing the hypothesis of germs.*

It would take too long to show you, how superficial he was in his experimentation. **No doubt, in the aftermath, the fox changed his mind!** *But who forced him to do so by making him come back from his mistake and his lightness? I'll tell you straightforwardly: it was me. In 1857, as a result of my experiments.*

In this letter : Antoine Béchamp does not simply accuse Louis Pasteur of plagiarism: he simply reproaches him for having understood nothing of the great discoveries of his century, and for having diverted them.

In 1854, I had verified the hypothesis of germs*, and concluded against spontaneous generation. I did not stop there, and from an uninterrupted series of works... the microzymian theory of living organization was complete in 1870, even from the point of view of pathology and therapeutics.*

A few years later, I had reduced the old germ hypothesis to its true proportions, by demonstrating that the so-called germs, are only the microzymas of extinct organisms.

I only add that pathology, according to the theory, that he admitted panspermia in the sense of my 1857 memoir, that is to say in the old sense, and took it upon himself to verify it, making the public, even the Academies, believe that by doing so he had victoriously fought against spontaneous generation.

I add, to refute your assertion that Pasteur had proved that every living being proceeds from a cell, that the famous microbist, in 1866-1867, when asked whether the cell was alive, pronounced himself in favor of the negative, **so that in 1876 he assured that the interior of the human** *body was comparable, with regard to the germs in the air, to the contents of a vase full of wine or beer.*

But where Pasteur's unconsciousness revealed itself most vividly was when in 1872 he tried to be credited, with the discovery of the facts of the microzyme theory, even from the pathological point of view.

Then he imagined what Dr. Roux called Pasteur's medical work, namely microbism, according to which, in addition to classical panspermia, there would be pathogenic panspermia.

Microbism is a monstrous fatalistic doctrine *since it supposes that at the origin of things God would have created the germs of microbes destined to make us sick. This is how the microcosm is the reverse forgery of the microzymian theory. This is to legitimize the expression of doer applied to your hero. I stop. Etc.*

Some courageous doctors have applied themselves, to unmasking the falsity of pastoral dogmatics. Thus they demonstrated, that microbes are generated in cells by degradation and recomposition, contrary to the Pasteurian dogma, which asserts that microbes are found in the air, in the virulent form found in a sick body.

Closer to home, Professor Jean Bernard asked the following question: ***"Are these viruses well outside of us? Are they not coming from our traumatized organisms?"*** As Hippocrates said: ***"The body makes a disease in order to cure itself".***

Like antibiotics, vaccines only diminish the vitality of the field, which diminishes natural resistance. This alteration of the soil may cause, cancer.

If doctors' demonstrations that vaccines do create a state of immune deficiency, were taken into account, then the governments, which obliges vaccination, would find itself in a very delicate position, with the risk of countless lawsuits.

One day, however, we will have to achieve this recognition, for lack of a complete disappearance of humanity as bees disappear, because of pesticides.

This would also be the end of the dogma of classical medicine. Officially, there is therefore no link between vaccines and the development of cancers, and other chronic diseases, and the question does not even deserve to be asked.

All immunologists agree, that immunity is still something that is extremely poorly understood. But immunology has little to say, in the face of the huge pharmaceutical market, represented by the massive vaccination of several billion individuals.

The 4 Pasteurian dogmas

1- When Pasteur finally understands that microbes exist in the air, he teaches that all microbes come from the air, and are the cause of diseases, the first dogma of the Pastorian religion, that of atmospheric panspermia.

2- Pasteur believes that every living being, protected from micro-organisms by its skin, is aseptic inside. Second pastoral dogma: that of the asepsis of living beings.

3- Pasteur believes that for each disease, the agent microbe is of a fixed, non-evolutive strain. This is the third pastoral dogma, that of microbial monomorphism. Béchamp discovers, for his part, that his microzymas, found in all living tissues, only separate from the organism and become morbid when the conditions of existence within the body fluids become precarious, that is to say abnormal. The composition of these liquids, which depends greatly on our diet and lifestyle, thus brings us back, to our individual responsibility in the face of disease.

4- Pasteur comes to consider external contamination as, the only source of infectious disease. For him, there is no doubt: microbial disease is given by the microbe, which is its agent, a perverse animal. It is the pastoral dogma of contagion that Béchamp rejects.

It is one thing to deny or pass over in silence the discoveries of his colleagues, to ridicule them, to affirm that his personal works are previous and when he cannot, to take on board the works he has ignored or criticized; **another thing is to understand nothing,** in the deepest sense of these experiences, and of the direction to be given to medicine.

This is Béchamp's accusation: he does not call Pasteur a criminal, but... It is therefore not essentially a claim of priority, even if it is clearly expressed: for these "microbes", which he will continue to call "microzymas" all his life, it is indeed he who discovered them and who knew how to show their origin, their action, their role in life and in illness, in the face of a **Pasteur, who understood nothing and was forced to build his work, on poorly digested recuperations.**

From the outset, he did not understand that the "figurative" ferments, which he called "globules", could come from other sources than air; nor did he understand the process of the act of fermentation by digestion of fermentable matter, passing through the action of a liquid, soluble ferment, a zymase, whose existence he always denied and whose name he never wanted to hear.

It was in 1907 that the German Büchner received the Nobel Prize for this invention!

The consequences of this misunderstanding, are extremely serious, since they have directly led modern medicine into a dead end, from which it will be very difficult to escape.

Professor Béchamp understood very well that gangrene, a microbial disease, comes from the decomposition of our organs by asphyxiation. It is enough to put a tourniquet around an arm or a leg, for several days to provoke this disease, without waiting for the action of some microbe of this disease in the atmosphere, where moreover one does not detect it.

Pasteur, convinced of the asepsis of the body, **comparing the body to a vase of wine or beer,** waits for an atmospheric microbe, to start fermentation, like putrefaction starts in a soup pot!

It is understandable that the therapeutics itself, based on one or the other of the two theories, is quite different.

The microbe is formed by the morbid evolution of the constituent microzymas, when the living conditions of these elements are no longer ordinary.

These morbid elements can then transmit the disease to other organisms, again if the conditions are favorable to receive them, it is clear. Personal and social responsibility are not escaped.

Remark by Professor Rappin: *"Let's remember what the study of the air has taught us, from a microbial point of view, namely that the air is always more or less loaded with germs, and in greater numbers the more we study it in inhabited environments, which could already lead us to suspect that if it is richer in microbes, in the most populated places, it is because the germs come from the organisms that live there...".*

Remark by the clinician and statistician Peter: *"Pasteur does not treat rabies, he gives it away!"*

The legend of Pasteur, could have quietly continued. For it is he who best described how evil microbes attacked poor humans. The discovery of microbes, fermentation, vaccination... it didn't take much to make Pasteur a national hero.

However, unluckily for him, in 1995, the scientific community wanted to commemorate the centenary of his death. Convinced biographers searched the archives.

Since then, other authors, such as Dr. Eric Ancelet, have systematically searched for the truth. The magazine Belle-santé relayed the serious doubts that historians and scientists, have recently expressed about Pasteur's inventions.

Pasteur has always been able to rely on the work of his contemporaries. This is normal for an open scientific mind. What is less so is that he has always managed to make us forget his predecessors.

Moreover, he used his high-ranking connections - and he could hardly go any higher since he was on the best terms with the wife of Napoleon III - to present "his" inventions and to further his career.

Pasteur relied on the work of Béchamp, Berthelot or even his collaborators whom he rarely cited. His own nephew, Adrien Loir, wrote: *"From day one, I became his thing, the indispensable accessory that he would use as he pleased, without finding resistance or contradiction."*

Doctor Eric Ancelet wrote: *"In 1878, Pasteur always fiercely denied the existence of enzymes, against the opinion of Marcellin Berthelot, Claude Bernard and Antoine Béchamp. Büchner will have the Nobel Prize in 1907 for this discovery of Béchamp. It will have taken 30 years to come back on a mistake!"*

Pasteur's work will not be understood, without recalling the historical environment of medical research at the time, the social issues of the second half of the 19th century when Pasteur published his work, and the character of the scientist.

It was a time when industry was draining rural emigrants to the suburbs. Misery, alcohol, unhealthy housing and dirt took hold of these populations. They are abandoned without resources as soon as illness or accidents strike them.

Pasteur agrees with some that the ills suffered by the unfortunate are due to an invisible agent. This is a godsend for the leaders of this society, who applaud and have applauded this providential find: **the occasional, apolitical and aconfessional microbe.**

As the hygienist movement develops (with Rudolf Virchow, Louis Kuhne, Sébastien Kneipp in Germany, Xavier Raspail in France, etc.), the gullible people are presented with their savior, a scholar before whom they kneel, author of indisputable works that make him, by eradicating their miseries, a benefactor of humanity, in the image of the Good Shepherd.

The microbes in the air

Pasteur will therefore develop a general theory that has resulted in several principles repeated and defended with energy:

- Our diseases come from microbes disseminated in the atmosphere.

- The microbe, like any other animal of creation, has similar parents.

- The higher animal and vegetable organisms are, in their interior, free of microbes. They defend themselves against their invasion and multiplication.

Pasteur's microbial theory has given medicine a special twist: **Pasteurism teaches us that we are victims of an external aggressor.**

Many voices were raised against this conception of life, seen "through the small end of a spyglass". Antoine Béchamp, of course, but later Jules Tissot, who showed that the bacillus Koch is the product of the degeneration of cells in diseased lung tissue; this ruined all pastoral conceptions and caused him a lot of trouble.

This demonstration demonstrates the complete uselessness of the BCG tuberculosis vaccine. Its dangerousness, on the other hand, is very real, which is **why German doctors have always been opposed to this vaccination,** which resulted in particular in the wearing of glasses for many schoolchildren entering the sixth grade, the period when vaccination was most often practiced.

VACCINATION AND RELIGION

Excerpts from the article published on October 8, 2015, by Michel Dogna, on the Alternative Santé website.

"The Faculty of Medicine of Geneva is today the temple and the seat of the dogma of vaccination, its new religion and its papess, Doctor Claire-Anne Siegrist. It is she who has been charged with launching a Europe-wide campaign to stop the nascent suspicion of vaccines as soon as possible, by not skimping on the means. The publicity kick-off was therefore

given on September 15, 2015 in Geneva with three conferences offered to the general public..."

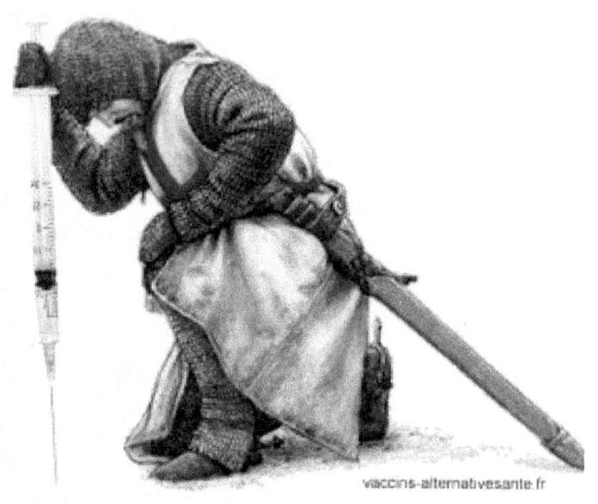

Let us recall the links that unite the Geneva Faculty of Medicine to the pharmas. Doctor Siegrist, a leading media expert, holds the chair of vaccinology at the Geneva Faculty of Medicine (the only one of its kind in Europe), created and subsidized by the Aventis-Pasteur laboratory, one of the largest vaccine manufacturers and supplier to the World Health Organisation.

Mrs. Siegrist talked about the most important of the four viruses, the vaccine hesitation, because for the moment no antidote has been found yet. It is highly contagious, represents 2 to 5% of the population, is spreading almost everywhere, and affects all social categories. They are sincerely convinced...

... She also said: *"Let's take a look at the successful strategy of the UK health service to get as many people as possible vaccinated against cervical cancer. Thanks to enormous advertising, which targeted doctors' surgeries, pharmacies, newspapers and schools, and also because public health officials went out to meet parents and teenage girls to convince them of the merits of this vaccine, the result was 93.5% vaccination coverage".*

... We are told that Switzerland is among the best performing countries in terms of health. Yet the health of adolescents is alarming: allergies, asthma, depression, anorexia, bulimia, hyperactivity, suicide... An article from the Swiss National Science Foundation alerts us: cancer is one of the main causes of death in children and adolescents! ***So, vaccination and cancer, simple coincidence?"***

The Bible to the rescue

In the United States, Jesse Johnson, on The Crippelgate website, published an article entitled "Anti-vaccination and epistemological narcissism", in which he appeals to Christian parents who are on the anti-vaccination side of the debate. The author mentions the recent measles epidemics in California and Arizona and blames anti-vaccination. The author implores Christian parents who choose not to vaccinate and, based on the Bible, gives **four reasons why Christians should vaccinate their children:**

1- "Vaccines are a common form of grace that has radically changed the world for the better (Genesis 3:18; Psalms 145:9-16; Matthew 5:44-45; Acts 14:16-17). Participating in the benefits of common grace in a post-Babelian society means that we bind ourselves together as a nation and use common grace to make the quality of life better (Genesis 9:6, 2 Kings 12:2, Luke 6:33). We work, we marry and we protect each other. A simple way to do this is to be vaccinated against diseases that plague crops that are not vaccinated.

2- Therefore, being vaccinated is a form of love for one's neighbor (Leviticus 19:18; Matthew 5:43, Romans 13:8-10, James 2:8). Knowing that some are too small, too young or too weak to be vaccinated, we protect the weak by being vaccinated.

3- We are not one of those who are influenced by the rumors on the internet which have since been widely discredited (Job 12:20; Proverbs 13:16). This does not mean that we blindly believe everything that "science" can say. Instead, we are endowed with a healthy skepticism that, in this case, is satisfied by the universal scientific call for the safety of these vaccines (coupled with its legal obligation in most states). In fact, our discernment is discredited when we believe unfounded rumors in the face of the obvious fact that measles once caused terror, which it no longer does today.

4- Christians are among those who take risks for the progress of the common good. We do not teach our children, "safety first" but rather "soli Deo Gloria" and everything else follows. Christians understood this in the past. The ethic of Jonathan Edwards, whose first act as president of Princeton was to receive a smallpox vaccine and later died from it, was the norm. The false ethic of Edwards' death is "avoid vaccines. The right moral is "take calculated risks for a better society."

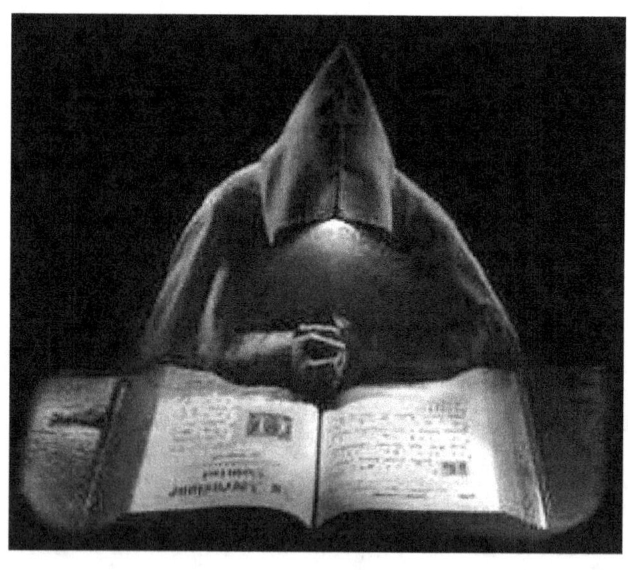

IS IT A SECT?

The frequent accusation of vaccination advocates who can't prove our arguments is to equate us with members of a sect. In order to see on which side cults are on, it therefore seems very instructive to pass the vaccination dogma through the filter of criteria generally defined by governments.

Definition: From an etymological point of view, the word "sect" would come from the Latin secta meaning the path one follows, party, cause, doctrine.

"A group of people who claim to be the same master and profess his philosophical doctrine and opinions."

"A group that follows a leader and is characterized by the fanaticism and intolerance of its members."

<u>Cults exercise real control over thought.</u>

Among the recognized criteria of sectarian aberration are the following:

- **mental manipulation,**
- **indoctrination,**
- **financial power,**
- **physical harm,**
- **the incontestability and infallibility of the doctrine,**
- **control of information sources,**
- **the cult of the guru's personality,**
- **attempts to infiltrate public authorities.**

With regard to these eight criteria, it is up to you, the reader, to judge which side the sectarians are on?

Mental manipulation

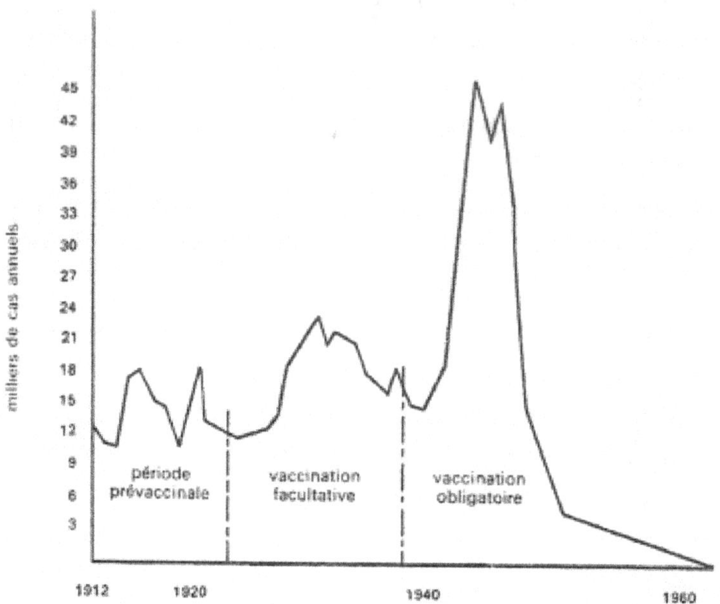

This is the graph of the evolution of diphtheria in France from 1912 to 1962, a period of 50 years. In France, during the pre-vaccination period, the average diphtheria rate was around 12,000 cases on average. From 1924 onwards, vaccination became increasingly widespread: the average rate was around 20,000 cases from 1924 to 1938.

In 1939-1940, vaccination became systematic and we then noted :

- 13,795 cases in 1940
- 46,750 cases in 1943
- 41,500 in 1944
- 45,500 in 1945

During these 5 years of mass vaccination, mortality was two to four times higher among the vaccinated than among the unvaccinated.

Including the year 1946, there were about 150,000 cases of diphtheria in addition to the usual number of cases before the vaccinations.

So, given these frightening statistics, how can proponents of vaccine orthodoxy claim that diphtheria vaccination has reduced the epidemic?

They present a graph on which the period during which vaccinations were carried out was staggered, a simple but **effective sleight of hand!**

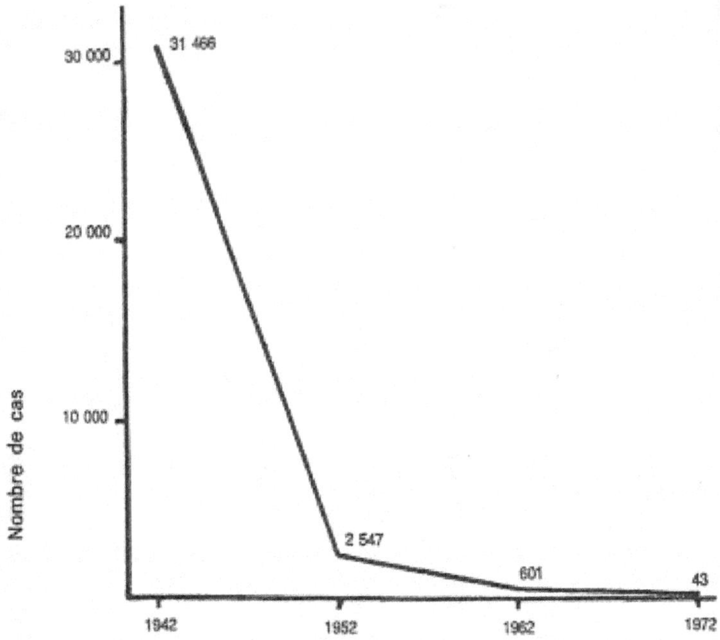

The figures reproduced above come from the then Minister of Health, Mr. Poniatowski. The top of the curve is taken immediately after its highest point, following the long vaccination campaign.

And what happened among an unvaccinated population? The following graph shows the number of cases and deaths in Scotland from 1941 to 1951.

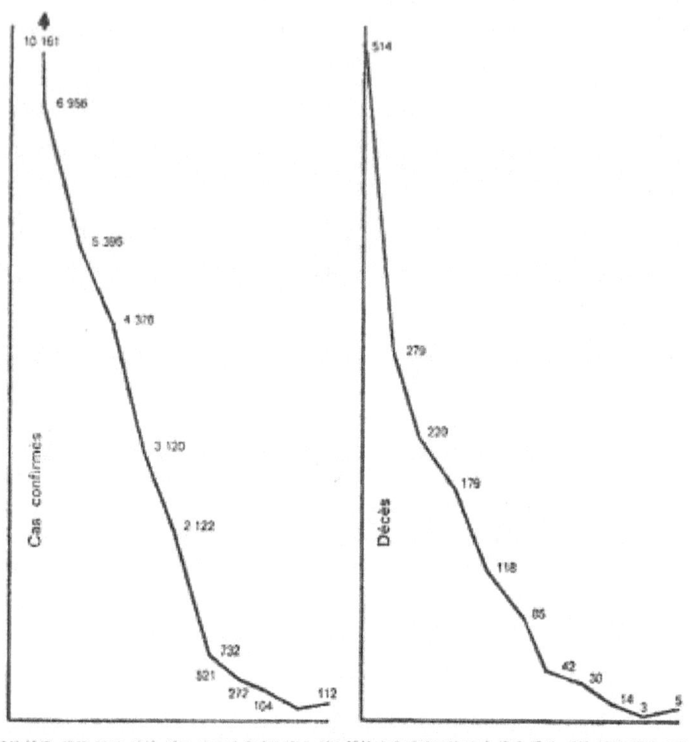

The graph above is an edifying demonstration of this. But there was also the manipulation of statistics, **moving a vaccinated population to a category of "inadequately or poorly vaccinated" and then to "unvaccinated".**

This was obviously to make the figures say the opposite of reality, as the number of sick people among the unvaccinated was lower than the number of vaccinated people! This is particularly to convince the public authorities to make the vaccination requirements a reality.

Result: vaccination seems to have dramatically reduced the epidemic. Which student could imagine being manipulated? And here he is now promoted as a defender of the vaccination dogma.

But there was also the manipulation of statistics, moving a vaccinated population to a category of **"inadequately or poorly vaccinated" and then to "unvaccinated".** This was obviously to make the figures say the opposite of reality, as the number of sick people among the unvaccinated is lower than the number of vaccinated people! This is particularly to convince the public authorities to make the vaccination requirements a reality.

An example: in Bonn, in 1871, there were 116 smallpox patients, 112 of whom were vaccinated and 4 unvaccinated. Among the latter, 2 died and 13 were vaccinated. Here is how

Official statistics were published: deaths among the non-vaccinated = 50%, deaths among the vaccinated = 12%.

These rates are mathematically exact, but without specifying the numbers of vaccinated and non-vaccinated, they make us believe in an enormous advantage in the vaccinated, with an obvious hecatomb in the non-vaccinated, **i.e. exactly the opposite of reality!**

The bigger it is, the bigger it gets: the last introduction of smallpox in France was by a soldier who was of course vaccinated. Well we did not hesitate to affirm that variolic viruses had been found,... **in the traveller's pajamas** (without specifying in which pocket)! The pirouette is of size: this man was vaccinated, therefore harmless, **but his pyjamas were not.** Quod erat faciendum.

Closer to home, during an endless flu vaccination campaign, the media all relayed this information: *"The virus is in Lyon, it should arrive in Marseille in two weeks."*

In other words, dear Provencal people, run to get the vaccine that will - it seems - be effective just as soon as the virus sets down its suitcases in the Phocaean capital!

Observers do not indicate the means of transport used by the bug, 20 kilometers a day, it must be a walker, a dog or a pigeon. In any case, it is for these birds that the "scientific" observers take us, not to say deep morons. Unfortunately their nonsense works, again and again for the same reason: **fear of disease.**

Indoctrination

The first force of indoctrination is ignorance. In France, at the beginning of the twentieth century there were, in our towns and countryside, three important people whose word was never questioned: the teacher, the priest and the doctor. All three were authoritative, notably because they had had long studies, unlike the majority of individuals.

Today, if the first two have seen their haloes collapse, the third has retained much of his influence on consciousness, at least in his field.

Thus, when a "vaccination heretic" tries to re-establish certain truths, he is immediately retorted: "You don't know what you are talking about, you didn't study medicine! " That's precisely why I can talk about it," replies the heretic, **"because your doctor doesn't even know about what I've learned!"**

Indoctrination consists of regularly using various means of psychological pressure such as fear, hope, guilt or the constant hammering of the same assertions, while attempting to short-circuit the critical thinking abilities of the person whose thoughts, or even personality, are to be changed.

"Son of a bourgeois or son of an apostle, all children are like yours, son of Caesar or son of nothing, all children are like yours... it's only afterwards, long afterwards... " These words from Jacques Brel's song illustrate a reality of all times: all children are the same at birth, and it is what is inoculated into their brains that will make them, either free spirits, or conditioned beings, and therefore slaves of thoughts that they could not question so much indoctrination has been, powerful.

As far as vaccination is concerned, indoctrination therefore begins at the earliest age, the age when adult teaching is never questioned. **Year after year, the seeds of lies are sown in each person's subconscious.** They will become almost indestructible certainties.

And no matter the age, social class or level of education, the indoctrinated person only reacts through his primitive brain: the cortex, considering any questioning of the vaccine dogma as a personal attack on its integrity. **The proof is that talking about the risks of vaccinations always triggers passionate and irrational reactions.**

And the extreme violence that sometimes verges on the hysteria of some supporters of vaccinations, against opponents shows to what extent their minds are no longer capable, of the slightest reasoning, as soon as the dogmas that have invaded their brains, are questioned to some extent.

For more than 150 years, the lies have not changed: regression of epidemics, harmlessness and protection against diseases. Who hasn't, at least once in his life, heard the nonsense of the rose thorn that can, for sure, give you tetanus. **Have you ever heard of any hecatomb among horticulturists?**

The act of vaccination has become so insignificant that it has even been illustrated in a proverb: "major and vaccinated".

There is, however, another that applies much better to this highly aggressive act: ***"Repeated 10 times, a lie is a lie. Repeated 1000 times, it becomes a truth."***

TV news " Soir 3 " of January 14, 2011, during a debate on drugs, a professor of medicine declared: ***" The training of the future doctor in pharmacology is null!"*** His colleague adds that, if he wants to complete his training, the medical student must do his own research.

Given the amount of work they have to do over many years, few students will add this extra research load.

Thus, every future member of the medical professions who has been indoctrinated with vaccines by parents, educators and the media since childhood is left in the dark about which substances he or she will order his or her patients to ingest.

Thus the future doctor, the future nurse, **become the loyal servants of the vaccine manufacturers.** And, as soon as he leaves the faculty, the young doctor is thus forced to contravene the Hippocratic oath he has just taken: ***"Primum, non nocere... First, do no harm..."***

The strongest argument of the Pasteurian religion, constantly repeated so that it takes deep root in the minds of all future inoculated: vaccination prevents millions of deaths. And many take this statement to the letter, without realizing its complete absurdity. Because, to put it plainly, it would mean that if 10 million people had not been vaccinated, those 10 million people would have died!

It is exactly the same absurd reasoning contained in this joke:

In Paris, every morning, a man spills a powder all around his vegetable garden. Intrigued after having seen this strange manege for 15 days, his neighbor asks him: *"But what is this powder that you pour every morning?"*. The man answered: *"It is anti-elephant powder."* The neighbor continues: *"But there are no elephants here."* And the man concludes, *"Of course, since I use powder!"*

As far as indoctrination is concerned, the Pasteurian religion has not invented anything, **it masterfully uses the best tool available: FEAR.** It seems that the memory of the great epidemics of the past centuries are inscribed in our genes. It is therefore not difficult, to convince us to receive pus injections by telling us that they protect us.

For example, the vaccination campaign for the fall of 2015: *"... to avoid hospitalization: get vaccinated..."* and to insist on the elderly who are *"... 3 times more at risk after the age of 65...".*

The older a person is, the more afraid they are of leaving their home and their loved ones for a hospital bed. Is playing on this fear humanly acceptable? Isn't this attitude equivalent to the dishonest walkers who take advantage of the weakness of our elders? The abuse of weakness is condemned by law... except for vaccine sellers?

And what about this 90-year-old man who, following his doctor's recommendations, got a flu shot and caught it in the days that followed? And what about his doctor's response to his patient's surprise, without the slightest analysis: "It wasn't the same virus! »

Financial power

To manufacture a product that every individual in a population is obliged to buy. **What could any industrial company dream of better?!** This product being, moreover, reimbursed by the Social Security...

Figures that stand on their own:

Vaccinations generate a worldwide turnover of 42.3 billion euros.

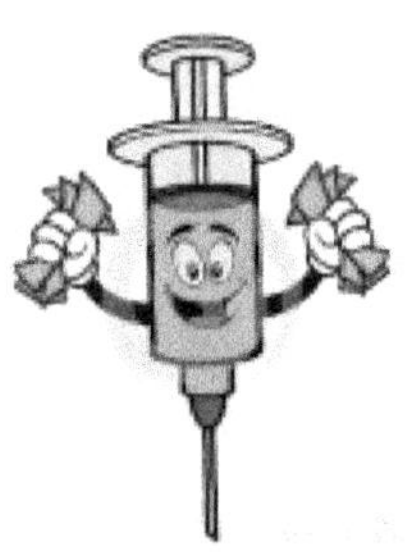

Violations of physical integrity

It is difficult to attack an individual's physical integrity more seriously than by forcing him to receive pus through a syringe! At the end of this book, you will hear a terrifying list of complications caused by vaccinations.

Incontestability and infallibility of the doctrine

To cast the slightest doubt on the efficacy and safety of vaccines immediately leads to being called irresponsible, ignorant, ideological, paranoid, crazy, dangerous to society.

Like its guru Pasteur, the strength of the vaccine religion and its leaders is that they have rallied the public authorities, regardless of the political color in place and the various ministers of health who have succeeded one another in all the republics since the invention of the vaccine.

They were thus able to pass the compulsory immunization laws, as described at the beginning of this book. Thus they turn the accusation of a cult against all those who challenge the doctrine, something that no physician would risk doing officially, at the risk of being purely and simply banned from practicing. Just like the student whose interest is not to study the texts of the detractors, at the risk of never obtaining his diploma.

Luckily we are not in a country where "re-education" camps exist, because there would be a few million of us locked up in them.

Control of information sources

Have you ever wondered why there has never been a major television or radio debate between proponents and opponents of vaccine dogmas?

First of all, because the vast majority of the media are indoctrinated on the subject.

Then because the ideological and simplistic arguments of the supporters of the vaccine dogma would come up against scientific facts, testimonies and real statistics provided by doctors qualified as heretics.

Yet vaccine manufacturers are not at all keen to see their sales skyrocket. Their pressure therefore nips in the bud any desire for such debates.

Cult of the personality of the guru

In France, how many hundreds of thousands of streets, avenues, boulevards and squares bear the name of the man who is almost described as the savior of humanity: Louis Pasteur? How many false books have been written about the man who himself lied about his alleged discoveries and alleged cures?

Yet it is said that the chemist, on his deathbed, acknowledged his errors. Too late, since he had already founded the institute that would bear his name and pursue his doctrine.

Attempts to infiltrate public authorities

How many public health decision-makers have more or less revealed links with the pharmaceutical industry?

This is the vaccine theory examined through the 8 criteria used to define a cult.

As with Galileo, will we have to wait another 200 years for the greatest medical aberration of the 20th century, perpetrated in the 21st century, to be recognized as such?

The facts are there, the proofs are there, in overabundance, unrecognized by official medicine, hidden from the eyes of the good "patients" who are fed lies and poisoned by pretending to protect them.

The main lie that serves as a basis for the vaccine doctrine: *"Vaccinations have caused epidemics to regress."* You will judge the truthfulness of this sentence by looking at the following graphs.

THE REGRESSION OF EPIDEMICS

Source: "L'intoxication Vaccinale" Fernand Delarue

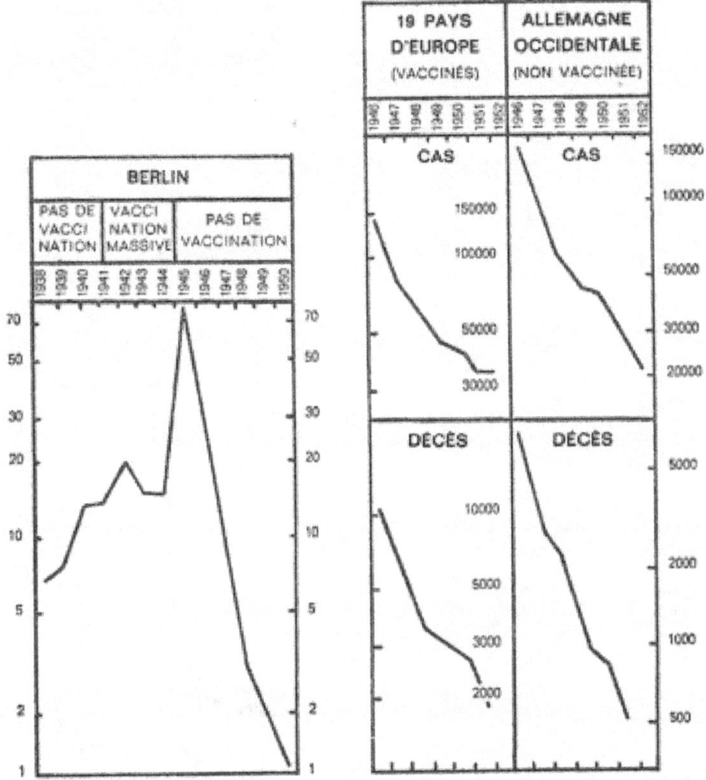

Graph on the left: Evolution of diphtheria in Berlin from 1938 to 1950. Mortality rate per 100,000 inhabitants. Logarithmic scale.

Right graph: Comparative decline of diphtheria in 19 vaccinated European countries and unvaccinated West Germany from 1946 to 1952. Logarithmic scale.

ANDRÉ HUAN

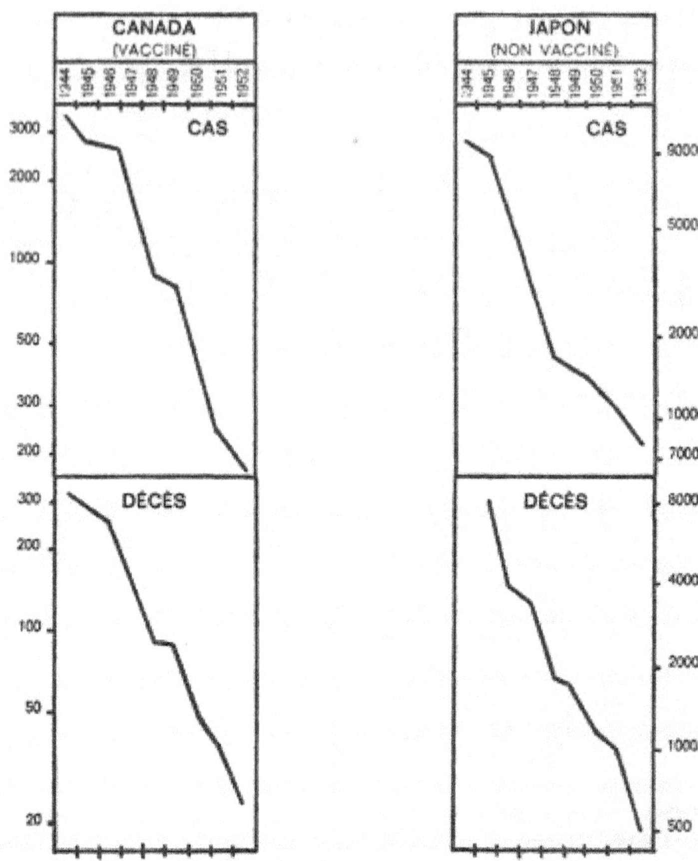

Comparative decline of diphtheria in vaccinated Canada and unvaccinated Japan from 1944 to 1952. Logarithmic scale.

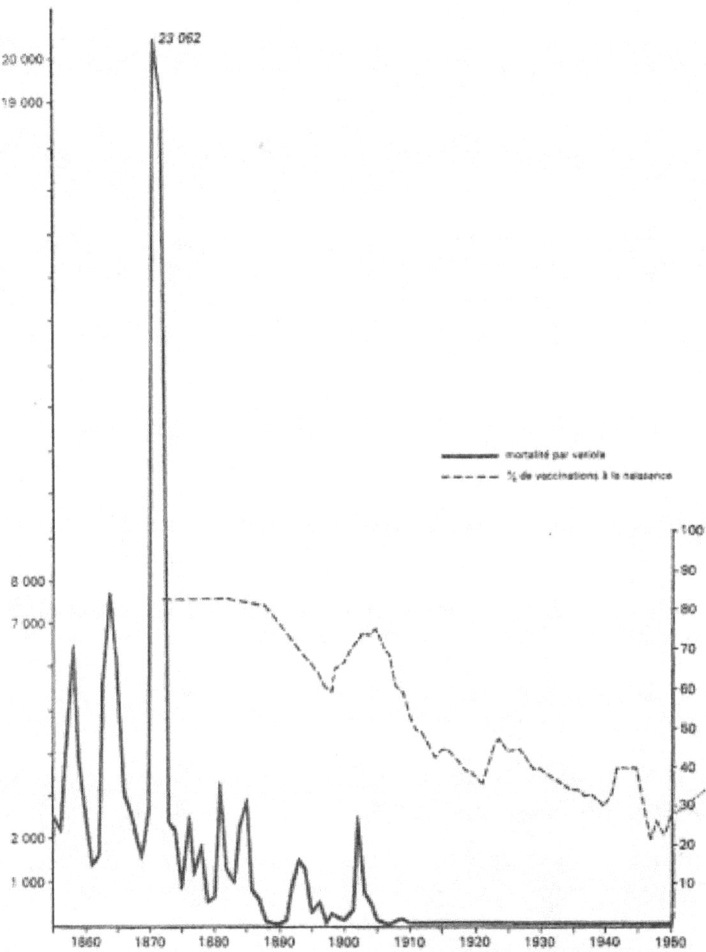

Mortality by smallpox (figures from the British Ministry of Health). 1853: vaccination becomes compulsory, 1867: prison sentences, seizures of property, 1875: law on public health (hygiene).

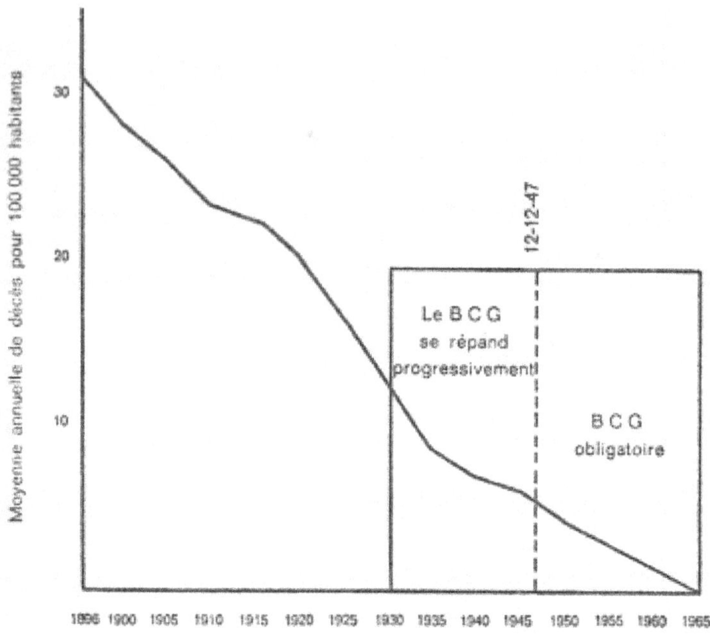

Decline of tuberculosis in Norway. As with diphtheria, only the boxed portion is retained, allowing the decline to be attributed to BCG.

Vaccination propaganda simply obscures the fact that tuberculosis had been declining sharply for 34 years without any vaccination.

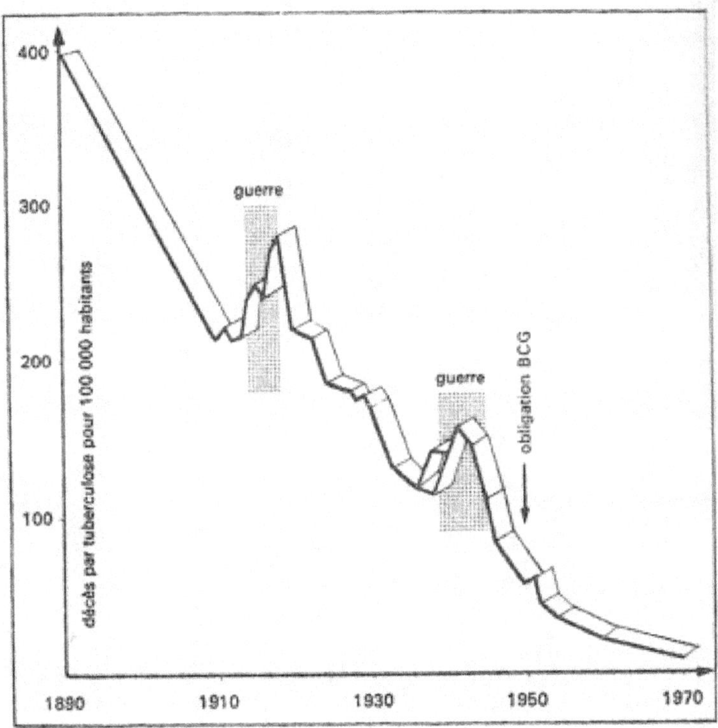

Evolution of tuberculosis mortality in France (INSERM figures). More than any other, this graph shows that when hygiene conditions are no longer satisfactory, which is always the case in times of war, diseases progress.

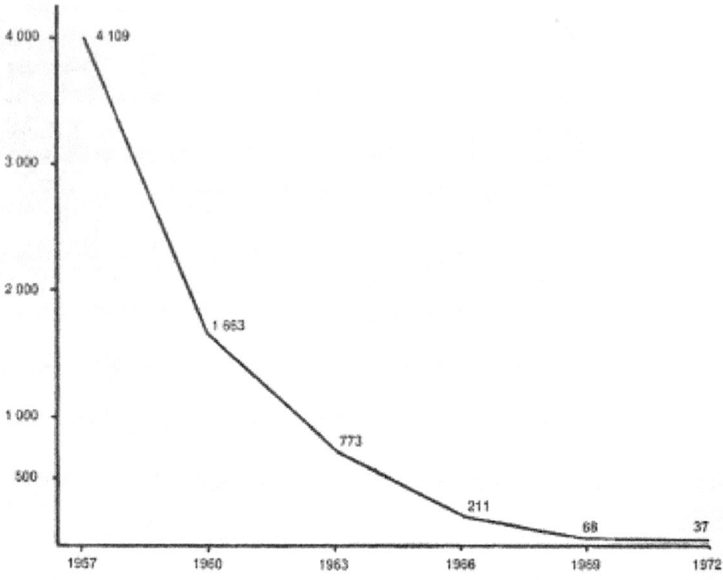

Decrease in polio cases, figures from Mr. Poniatowski, then Minister of Health. The same figures are presented in the following graph, in dot-dashes.

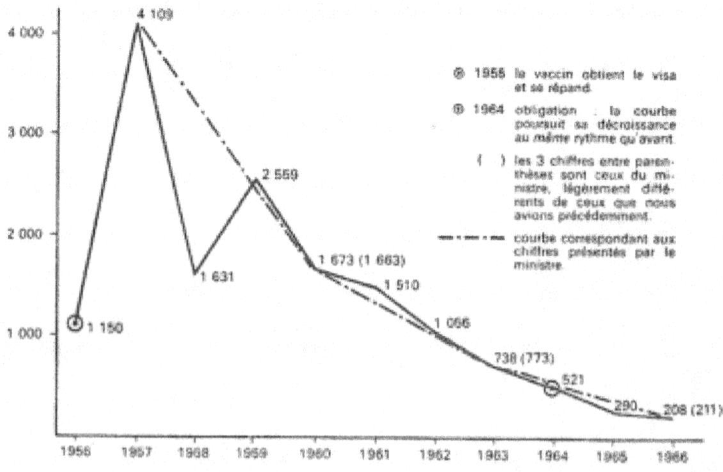

Again, as with diphtheria and tuberculosis, the manipulation is obvious, as the Minister takes 1957 as the starting point, while the vaccine was being spread from 1956 onwards, causing an unprecedented rise in the number of cases.

And since it is always good to look at the curve of the disease over the longest possible period, the following graph is even more telling.

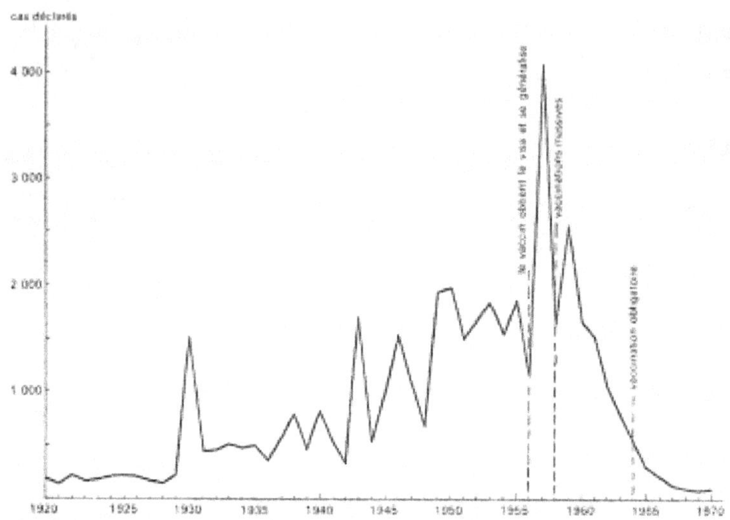

As shown above, from 1962 onwards the curve continues the decline that began in 1955 before vaccination. And the 1964 vaccination obligation in no way affects the regression.

As we have just seen in these various graphs, **the fact that vaccination has caused an epidemic to decline is not at all demonstrated, quite the contrary.**

This is, however, the main false argument used by the vaccine religion to justify its practices.

A convincing example is that of smallpox, for which the WHO had to stop its mass vaccination campaigns with catastrophic results and replace them with simple isolation measures that alone succeeded in eradicating the epidemic.

That's how smallpox disappeared, and vaccines had nothing to do with it, except to have forced hundreds or thousands of children to spend their entire lives curled up in wheelchairs as a result of post-vaccine encephalitis caused by this supposedly harmless injection.

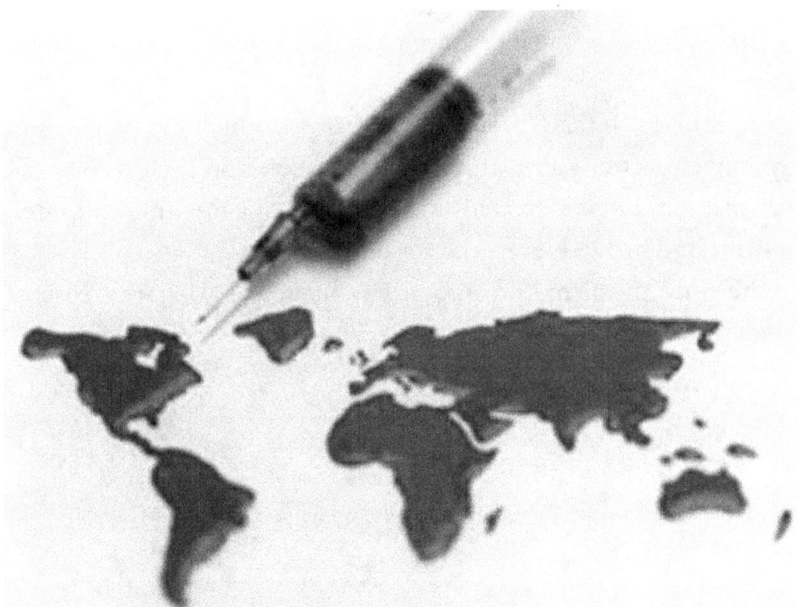

Diphtheria - Tetanus – Poliomyelitis

These are the 3 vaccines among the 11 that are still mandatory in France.

Diphtheria, Tetanus and Poliomyelitis for which the vaccine is not only dangerous but above all totally ineffective and useless since these three diseases can be treated and cured by magnesium chloride, as demonstrated by Dr. Neveu and his disciples.

The only problem for laboratory finances is that the cost of a treatment with magnesium chloride is absolutely derisory (around $1).

DIPHTERY

Auguste Neveu was born on the island of Oleron in 1885. He studied at the Faculty of Medicine of Bordeaux where he graduated at the top of his class. After serving in the navy as a medical officer, which earned him the Legion of Honor, he opened a practice in his native department of Charente-Maritime, in Rochefort.

Married then to a resident of the village near Breuil-Magné, he settled there, and as was often the case at that time, country doctors were also solicited by their patients to treat animals.

Dr. Neveu, having had knowledge of Professor Delbet's publications at the Academy of Medicine, experimented in 1932 with the use of magnesium chloride to treat a calf suffering from foot-and-mouth disease and a dog with distemper, sometimes called "dog polio".

When the calf and the dog were cured, **Dr. Neveu began treating his patients' infectious diseases with magnesium chloride,** curing bronchitis, pleurisy, angina and childhood diseases.

It was then that the terrible flu epidemic of the winter of 1935, known for its serious bronchopneumonic complications, occurred. Dr. Neveu's patients were cured thanks to magnesium chloride, and conversely, his colleagues' flu patients were cured in the classic way, **and his reputation spread throughout the region.**

Encouraged by his results, he successfully extended the prescription of magnesium chloride to other diseases, particularly diphtheria and poliomyelitis, which were devastating at that time.

June 14, 1944

My dear colleague,

The office of the Academy of Medicine makes incredible and unforeseen difficulties to let me present your work on your behalf.

By regulation, any work that is not a member of the Academy must be submitted to the Board in advance. I have therefore sent yours to the said Council. Usually this is a simple formality. Up to now, I have never encountered any difficulties.

But yesterday I was informed that your work had to be submitted to some health commission. I could see there only a delaying tactic intended to prevent or at least to delay the publication...

I stated that I would make the communication on my behalf and that I intend to make it next Tuesday. I don't know if I will be successful

June 20, 1944

A violent, almost dramatic, unique scene has just taken place at the Academy of Medicine. I have written you all the adventures that preceded the inclusion on the agenda of my communication, or rather yours.

Finally I was on the agenda. But at the beginning of the session the president declared that he could not give the floor to a communication on the treatment of diphtheria with magnesium chloride.

After a long and painful public discussion, I got to read what I had written. So I did a reading - but the president said that the board reserved the right to ban it from publication and that he would notify his decision next Tuesday.

You can see that I was right to think that the board wanted to filibuster. My communication is worded in such a way that I find it difficult to refuse its inclusion in the newsletters. However, you can expect anything from people with such a bias.

November 16, 1944

My dear colleague,

... The publication of my communication of June 20th is definitively refused. The Board of the Academy found after six months of reflection the following argument: by making known a new treatment for diphtheria, one would prevent vaccinations and the general interest is to generalize these vaccinations.

The Board had the pretension of not even mentioning my communication in the bulletin. I protested strongly. My communication having been read in public session, the title should appear in the bulletin.

I asked that after the title, it be indicated that the publication had been refused. I could not get satisfaction on this last point. This is very significant. They are refusing publication, but they don't want to take responsibility for the refusal.

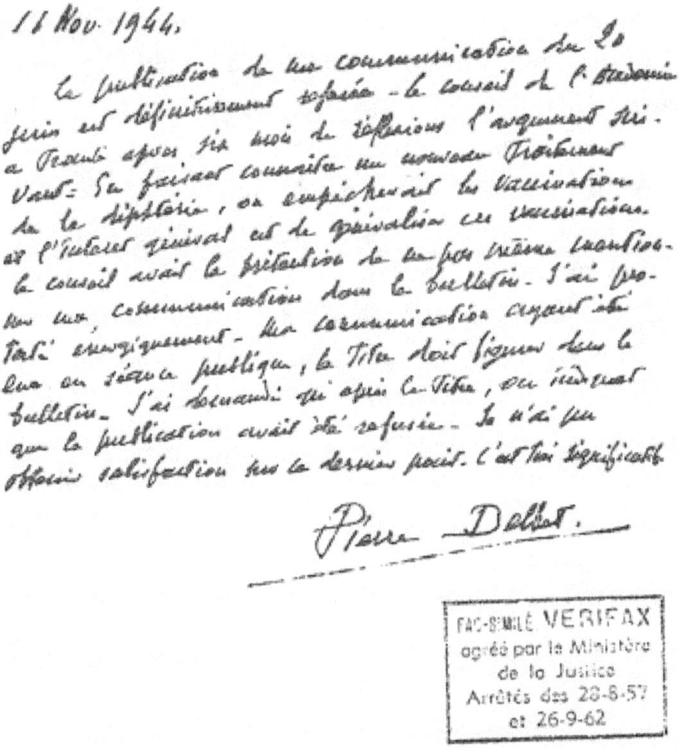

11 Nov. 1944.

[handwritten letter in French, signed] Pierre Delbet.

Unbelievable admission from the Academy! Hard to find a more dazzling testimony! This is how the leaders of the Pasteurian religion stifled a treatment, that could have saved thousands of children but would have harmed the sale of vaccines. When it comes to ensuring the success of vaccinations, **it doesn't matter that thousands of lives are at stake.** This proves what powerful interests dictated its conduct at the Academy of Medicine at the time.

Even worse, although Dr. Neveu found that magnesium chloride also cured polio within 48 hours from 1943 onwards, when administered at the onset of the first symptoms, he never managed to spread his method.

This was at the time of the launch of the French polio vaccine. As this event is always supported by an overwhelming media campaign that brandishes the threat of death, the trembling public was immediately convinced to switch to injections.

But what would have happened to the vaccination if the French had learned that the disease, taken at its onset, could be cured more easily than a head cold and without leaving any after-effects?

We know the answer: the laboratories would have had to forego hundreds of millions of dollars in sales.

The cures obtained with magnesium chloride treatment (cytophylactic method), although published in a brochure by Dr. Neveu, never appeared in any medical society journal. Worse, Professor Lépine did not hesitate to lie to divert from this method all those who might be interested in it.

Thus he published the following article in the Republic of the Center, then in the Lausanne Gazette on June 10, 1959: *"To affirm to families that they could, when the time came, cure poliomyelitis with a simple method (administration of a magnesium salt) when the total inefficiency of this method is amply demonstrated, constitutes pure and simple moral swindle."*

Through the intermediary of Henri Geffroy, founder of La Vie Claire, Mr. Clerc then proposed that the debate be decided by an honorary jury, composed of half of doctors chosen by both parties. A certain number of polio patients could thus be selected, accepted without contest by each member of the jury, and Dr. Neveu would treat them.

If he failed, this failure would be published and his method, recognized as illusory and erroneous, would sink into oblivion. But if he succeeded in curing polio as he claimed, then his success would have to be publicized everywhere, so that no patient would be deprived of his chances of recovery.

Dr. Neveu replied by return of mail that this was his greatest wish and that he was ready to undergo the test. But Professor Lepine denied that he had made any accusation against Dr. Neveu, claimed to have experimented with the method in his laboratory, and refused the honorary jury, considering **"any further experimentation to be superfluous."**

To say that it is such attitudes that have shaped today's medicine, flouting Science as it is not allowed!

Even today, researchers, professors and doctors from all over the world are insulted and called ideologues when they want to demonstrate the danger of vaccinations, **thereby putting their careers in danger.**

But aren't all ideologists blindly following the erroneous dogmas of an obscurantist chemist who believed in spontaneous generation, of a thief who understood absolutely nothing about the discoveries he stole?

And if we are ideologues, why not seize the opportunity of great televised debates to make fools of us all in good faith and thus bring back to reason all those who doubt the benevolence of vaccines? So what would scientists fear in the face of ideologues? **What would they be afraid of?**

TETANOS

Logically, Dr. Neveu thought that the simplest method to destroy an anaerobic is to send him a lot of oxygen, especially with a powerful oxygenant: magnesium.

Collaborator of Dr. Neveu, Dr. Chavannon, chief physician at the Paris hospitals published this report: *"The terminal man was revolted as a spring blade on a table with the trismus of the jaw, and breathing was short. I gave him an intravenous injection with 5 g of magnesium chloride dissolved in 20 ml of saline; the injection was carried out in 20 minutes (1 ml per minute). A few minutes after the injection was completed, the man relaxed and sat down quietly; he asked me for a cigarette and stood up."*

Like diphtheria or polio, tetanus can be cured even in the terminal phase. But beware of the doctor who would apply this treatment, there is a strong risk that he could be suspended for 6 months at best for "breaching protocol", as was the case a few years ago, for a practitioner in Finistère.

Outside the medical profession, few people know that tetanus can be a victim of tetanus several times, i.e. the disease itself does not immunize. Professor Tissot, a true scientist, asked the right question: ***"Since a patient cured of tetanus is never immune to a second attack, how could a vaccine better protect against the disease?"***

Moreover, tetanus being a non-contagious disease, there can be no contamination and therefore no epidemics. So what is the interest, apart from that of laboratories, to vaccinate an entire population of infants?

Let's go further, in order to prove that a toxoid is protective, we need to do experiments. **Well, only one was enough,** conducted by Gaston Ramon, to establish that the vaccine was effective. He administered a high dose of tetanus toxin to rabbits, and then injected them with a dose of tetanus toxoid. Because the rabbits survived, he concluded, that the vaccine was protective.

He simply forgot, that the toxin emitted by the bacillus does not circulate in the blood (aerobic environment). By injecting the toxin, he made it circulate in the blood, where it actually encountered antibodies generated by the toxoid.

However, during tetanus disease, the toxin remains in the anaerobic wound, and is then propelled into the nerve pathways, which are inaccessible to the antibodies.

To say that the vaccine is immunizing is a huge lie, a medical deception, that no one has ever caught, allowing mass vaccination of adults and children.

Although it has long since disappeared from industrialized countries, tetanus in newborns persists in some countries where hygiene is non-existent. China has been able to reduce neonatal tetanus deaths by 90% thanks to the "3 C's" strategy: clean hands, clean cord, clean delivery table.

But instead of promoting hygiene education, World Health Organisation advises and supports mass vaccination campaigns.

A particularity of the anti-tetanus vaccine revealed by an experiment carried out in Vienna (Austria) in 1984: **it weakens the immune system.** A simple anti-tetanus booster is capable of unbalancing the ratio between CD4 and CD8 lymphocytes (those involved in AIDS) on about the 14th day after the injection.

There are dogmas that have a hard life, that of the tetanus vaccination is one of the most unbreakable. *"If there is a vaccine to be made, it is the tetanus vaccine,"* is the language of medical orthodoxy, which has the support of the majority of the population.

The notion of microbial polymorphism defended by Professor Béchamp, was taken up by Professor Jules Tissot at the beginning of the 20th century. He hypothesized that the tetanus bacillus, Clostridium tetanii, would result from the transformation of the E. coli Escherichia coli, that colonizes the intestines of humans and mammals, making tetanus an endogenous disease. This would explain why burn victims, can develop tetanus.

Magnesium chloride is immuno-stimulant because it helps in the formation of antibodies, it is anti-infectious by stimulating phagocytosis, it is restorative because it blocks the proliferation of germs, it is also a nerve regulator, by normalizing the excitability of nerves, a natural sedative and anti-depressant and finally a general stimulant for the body, because it increases the resistance and activity of cells.

Françoise Joët writes in her book: Tetanus: the mirage of vaccination :

"In 1959 Edsall already spoke of the failure of the vaccine. Goulon in 1972 saw 10 out of 64 vaccinated patients contracting tetanus. The same thing happened with Berger in 1978, who noted various observations of well-vaccinated patients who had nevertheless contracted tetanus.

Passen and Andersen in 1986 cite the case of a 35-year-old man who had contracted tetanus despite an antibody level 16 times higher than the threshold considered protective. He had received all the recalls in his childhood and all the regular recalls up to 4 years before the accident.

Crone and Reder in 1992 describe 3 patients who developed severe tetanus despite high antibody titration. One of these patients died. Two of them had been vaccinated one year before contracting the disease. One had been deliberately hypervaccinated in order to commercially produce tetanus globulin.

Very interesting also this observation collected in Finland: from 1969 to 1985, 106 cases of tetanus were reported...66% were vaccinated....

All vaccinations, including tetanus vaccination, have been found to cause bastard forms of the disease, with confusing symptoms and a pathological condition of difficult description.

Magnesium chloride is certainly the product that most successfully cures tetanus, as well as other infectious diseases such as diphtheria, poliomyelitis...".

POLIOMYELITIS

Since the disease disappeared from Europe in 2002, why should we continue to be vaccinated? This is also the case throughout the American continent and in the Western Pacific, including China.

To justify the continuation of the vaccination program, we are told that we must "eradicate the virus from the surface of the planet." **As if man can eradicate a virus!** Viruses are everywhere and the polio virus is still there. **The circulation of the wild virus remains the best protection since its presence in our intestines makes us naturally immune.**

Of course, the argument is made that "vaccination coverage" would protect the community. However, this argument is totally false!

It is perhaps in 1956 that this hypothesis was made sacred, by the declaration that Mr. Poniatowski made in Chatou: *"If you vaccinate the entire child population, beyond 85%, you break the chain of contagion and there is no longer any spread of the virus... If you do not vaccinate children, they become carriers of the virus that they spread around them."*

Although this theory is appealing, it is not at all corroborated by the facts. The example of Great Britain is a vivid demonstration of this. Faced with the failure of smallpox vaccinations, this country gradually stopped vaccinating, hence the prophecy of the vaccination community of an imminent catastrophe.

In 1925, Bernard Shaw, the great opponent of vaccinations, described how triumphantly impatient the proponents of vaccination were awaiting the arrival of the next epidemic, since the proportion of those vaccinated had fallen to 40%. And it is the opposite that happens: not only is there no epidemic, **but smallpox regresses until it disappears completely, in a country that is less and less vaccinated!**

In 1949, all compulsory laws were repealed and freedom was once again granted to British citizens, and in 1973, the British Minister of Health advised against vaccination when immunization coverage was less than 5%, which in no way led to the return of an epidemic.

But it must be believed that, as with the Chernobyl cloud that stopped at our border, it is quite different in France, since in 1975 the Minister of Health declared to the National Assembly: *"It is necessary to continue the practice of vaccinations, because the circulation of germs persists and we observe that epidemics reappear as soon as the overall immune coverage of the population decreases."*

But let's go back to polio, where, when a few cases resurface in India or Africa, we are told that it is due to insufficient vaccination, whereas there is massive vaccination thanks to Unicef, Rotary or the Bill Gates Foundation.

In Holland, in 1978 and 1992, the extremely rare infectious outbreaks were attributed to sects opposed to vaccination. In truth, the majority of its members **were duly vaccinated** and no cases were found among the 400,000 people who were not vaccinated for reasons other than religious ones.

The truth is that there are multiple counter-examples (Oman, Finland, Israel...) showing that polio restarts after vaccination campaigns or that it develops in vaccinated populations.

In two cases (Madeira Island in the 1960s and Albania in the 1990s), the coincidence between the arrival of the vaccine and the return of polio was absolutely flagrant.

In France, the number of deaths among those affected exploded from 1964, the date of compulsory vaccination.

Like many vaccines, the development of polio caused heavy human losses. The Salk vaccine, in particular, was responsible for a veritable hecatomb in 1955 in California: 220,000 people were infected, 70,000 were sick, 164 were severely paralyzed, and at least 10 died.

For other vaccine preparations, disabled people, prisoners, and African children were used as guinea pigs. Cultivated on monkey kidneys, Sabin oral vaccine was tested on 80 million people. What was not known at the time was that it contained retroviruses very similar to HIV, the AIDS virus.

Polio always occurs when hygiene conditions are poor, such as when there is no sewage or running water. Its disappearance is most likely due to the development of drinking water supply and sanitation systems. As the virologist Peter Duesberg likes to ironise, the victory over infectious diseases is more the work of plumbers than doctors.

In Western countries today, there are hardly any vaccine-induced polio diseases left in the world. And in the Third World, sensitivity to wild viruses has clearly increased as a result of polio vaccinations.

True polio prophylaxis is based on simple hygiene measures and the abandonment of vaccination. And when the disease breaks out, there is still a cure. The biggest lie by omission of the vaccine propaganda: Polio is incurable, when on the contrary it is easily fought.

There are three ways to fight polio:

- Dr. Nephew's, using magnesium chloride,

- That of Dr. Fred R. Klenner who, in 1948, in North Carolina, used vitamin C in massive injections (several tens of grams per day) on 60 patients who all recovered without sequelae in 3 to 5 days. He made his method known at the annual meeting of the American Medical Association and later published several articles on the subject, but the lack of interest from the scientific press and authoritative specialists in the field at a time when everyone was thinking more about the possibility of vaccination, meant that he was little followed and his method fell into oblivion.

- Dr. Pilette's method, which suggests a supplement of iodine. In the 1950s, several doctors successfully tested this type of treatment because polio seemed to be more prevalent in countries with no access to the sea, such as Switzerland and Austria. Like magnesium chloride and vitamin C, however, the marine trace element was swept away by the invention of various vaccines, which were much more cost-effective than non-patentable molecules.

In conclusion, if these three methods have fallen into oblivion, it is because pharmaceutical companies have no interest in exploiting them.

If you are curious, ask your doctor if, in the course of his or her long studies, he or she has heard about these methods and their inventors. If not, he or she is one of the victims of misinformation and the thirst for profit continues to threaten all children with DTP, a dangerous, useless and ineffective vaccine.

SUDDEN INFANT DEATH SYNDROME

Sudden Unexplained Infant Death Syndrome (SIDS) is the sudden death of an infant that occurs unexpectedly and for which complete postmortem examinations cannot reveal a precise cause of death. Most commonly, it is an infant between 2 and 4 months of age who is found dead in his or her crib.

In his book **"Vaccination, Social Violence and Criminality- The Medical Assault on the American Brain"** (1990), Harry L. Coulter, medical historian, writes :

"We estimate that at least 1,000 babies die each year from this vaccine (DTP), while 12,000 children become disabled for life. Our figures have never been challenged by the medical establishment... This program continues every day, hundreds of perfectly healthy babies are thus transformed into deficient beings: mentally retarded, blind, deaf, epileptic, infirm, unstable, future delinquents, proven criminals. All this may seem terribly exaggerated; however, these are serious and moderate conclusions based mainly on the evidence accumulated in the following pages... Any vaccination is likely to cause mild or severe encephalitis... If some foreign enemy had inflicted such damage on the country, a declaration of war would have immediately followed...".

Harry L. Coulter wrote 1,000 babies in 1990 and it's 2021. Given the staggering increase in the number of immunization campaigns, that number of 1,000 babies must, alas, be greatly multiplied today.

Already in 1970, Dr. Archie Kalokerinos, from the Biological Research Institute in Australia, and his colleague Dr. Glen Dettmann discovered a clear link between immunological deficiency caused by vaccination and sudden and unexplained infant death syndrome.

On May 24, 1987, Dr. Kalokerinos sounded the alarm in the Sunwell Tops newspaper about the pertussis vaccine: ***"It's the worst of all. It is responsible for a large number of deaths and irreversible brain damage in newborns."***

After years of observation, the Australian Viera Scheibner, with the help of her engineer husband, developed a monitoring device capable of monitoring the breathing of infants to prevent sudden death. In her book "Vaccination", published in 1993, she demonstrated the responsibility of the DTPoq vaccine in this syndrome.

However, in the March 25, 1995 Medical Competition, Dr. P. Touze dared to write: *"[...] I believe that we must stop blaming vaccines for the occurrence of unexplained cot death. This is bad for the morale of the vaccinated population... and for the vaccinators."* **For this doctor, infant death is less important than the morale of the vaccinators. It's up to you to judge.**

Michael Belkin, President of Belkin Limited, a global investment firm, is a prominent businessman in the United States. Since the death of his little girl at five weeks of age, 15 hours after she received her second injection of hepatitis B vaccine in September 1998, he has been dedicated to finding the real cause of her death and the lies of his country's health care organizations, which have nothing to envy ours.

He was shocked by the autopsy report. The New York coroner ruled that it was MSIN, but neglected to mention in his report that the baby had swelling of the brain and that she had just received the Hepatitis B vaccine, even though on the day of the autopsy the coroner had confirmed that the brain was enlarged.

"Through multiple discussions with other experienced pathologists, I later discovered that swelling of the brain is a classic side effect of vaccination (with any vaccine) in the medical literature."

On November 3, 1973, the French magazine La Gazette médicale admitted: **"It is because the risk of post-vaccination neurological accidents is higher than that of death or encephalopathic damage due to whooping cough itself, that the Swedes and Germans no longer advocate this vaccination and that the Proffessor Gordon Steward multiplied communications and interventions so that English babies are no longer exposed to it."**

But French babies do not have the chance to benefit from the same protective measures! The Germans have finally removed the generalized vaccination against whooping cough from their vaccination schedule. For them, the regression of whooping cough has nothing to do with vaccination, which is more dangerous than non-vaccination.

Professor Ehrengut, who has been studying the complications of vaccination for 35 years, believes that they are largely underestimated (Quick-Nachrichten No. 51 of December 11, 1975).

By delaying vaccination against pertussis after the age of two years, the Japanese have noted a very significant decrease in sudden and unexplained infant death, which would prove that the vaccine does indeed play a role in the syndrome (J. D. Cherry "Pertussis vaccine encephalopathy" Jama - 1990).

Here are two tables from a report by the British laboratories GSK (GlaxoSmithKline).

The first table concerns deaths collected after Infanrix Hexa vaccinations between October 23, 2010 and October 22, 2011.

Case Number	Age of the vaccinated child	Number of doses received prior to death	Time from last dose to death
1	2 months	1	12 days
2	2,5 months	1	1 day
3	9 months	2	102 days
4	10 months	2	1 day
5	2 months	1	1 day
6	11 months	3	3 days
7	5 months	2	1 day
8	18 months	?	1 day
9	1,5 months	1	14 hours
10	3 months	1	5 days
11	3 months	2	1 day
12	2,5 months	1	2 days
13	5 months	2	1 day (30 hours)
14	3 months	1	8 days

Case Number	Age of the vaccinated child	Number of doses received prior to death	Time from last dose to death
1	4 months	3	11 days
2	3 months	2	2 days
3	2 months	?	21 days (first signs within 24 hours)
4	3,5 months	?	4 days
5	1 month + 3 weeks	1	4 days
6	2 months	1	5 days (first signs within 12 hours)
7	6 months	3	5 months (first signs within 5 days)
8	3 months	?	11 days
9	3 months	1	3 days
10	3 months	2	9 days
11	3 months	1	1 day
12	3 months	1	1 day
13	2 months + 1 week	1	3 days
14	?	?	?
15	2 months	1	1 day
16	11 mois	1	1 day
17	6 months	3	9 days
18	2 months	1	12 hours
19	4 months	1	1 day
20	5 months	3	3 days
21	5 months	3	less than 1 day
22	3 months	1	7 days

The second of the deaths collected after Infanrix Hexa vaccinations between October 23, 2009 and October 22, 2010, (i.e. a total of 14 + 22 = 36 deaths over a period of 2 years).

It should be remembered that only 1 to 10% of serious side effects of vaccines are actually identified and recorded according to official medical journals.

Infanrix™ hexa

Summary Bridging Report

Date of the Report: 16 December 2011

International Birthdate: 23 October 2000 (European Union)

Data Lock Points : 23 October 2009 to 22 October 2011

Author	
Vanessa Coremans, Safety Scientist	
Signature	Date
Reviewer	
Dr. Felix Arellano, MD Vice President, Head Biological Clinical Safety and Pharmacovigilance, GlaxoSmithKline Biologicals	
Signature	Date

ASTHMA AND ALLERGIES

It was the Austrian paediatrician Clemens Von Pirquet who first used the term "allergy" at the end of the 19th century. Working on mice, he showed that mice died quickly after a second injection of egg protein. He also observed that patients who had received injections of horse serum or a smallpox vaccine reacted more quickly and more severely after a second injection.

He suggested the term "allergy" from the Greek words allos (other) and ergon (reaction) for this hypersensitivity reaction. The Greek word "anaphylaxis" or "atopy" is also used.

Any allergy is caused by an internal disorder; it is the result of an over-reaction of an organism in a state of adaptive incapacity, leading to an inadequate immune response.

In addition to the chemical substances that invade our environment, the main cause of allergies comes from over-vaccination. **Allergy is nothing more than a malfunctioning of our immune system.** One of the most frequently mentioned effects is angioedema: the vaccine allergy shock causes the face to swell and disrupts breathing and swallowing.

In addition, in vaccinated mothers, the foetus is unable to build up an intestinal flora rich in protective endogenous bacteria, resulting in a propensity to allergies later on, anywhere in the world (Lancet, April 7, 2001).

In countries with a high incidence of vaccination, the number of allergies is growing by more than 10% per year. 30% of children aged 6-7 and 40% of adolescents are affected.

Different allergies: eczema, asthma or hay fever can coexist, not to mention the many food allergies that are the sixth leading cause of illness in the world.

Vaccinations destabilise the field and weaken the immune system, which then allows tolerance to pathogens, and above all a transformation of acute diseases into chronic ones.

Published in the journal Science, a study carried out in Japan on 867 children who received BCG and tuberculin tests. 36% of the children followed developed allergies, including severe forms of asthma.

On the other hand, a number of studies have pointed out that childhood diseases, which we want to eradicate at all costs, play a vital role in strengthening the immune defences and consolidating the ground and protect against certain pathologies, particularly allergies.

The first BCG Congress unanimously confirmed that BCG causes a clear and long-lasting allergy, detected by tuberculin, within a short period of time. Among unvaccinated children, Swedish researchers found a 3% allergy frequency to tuberculin, while vaccinated children had an allergy frequency of 49%, well above the expected maximum of 7.8%.

The mumps vaccine induces many allergies, particularly to egg proteins and the neomycin it contains.

As for the hepatitis B vaccine, it promotes allergies, eczema, urticaria and angioedema, which suggest the possible role of vaccine adjuvants.

According to an Anglo-Saxon study by Oxford's Churchill Hospital, **the significant increase in asthma, which has doubled in France** in the last twenty years with 3,500 deaths per year, is more related to vaccines, particularly BCG and the vaccines against whooping cough and measles, than to pollution.

A study published by the journal Science in 1997 showed that asthma accounted for two thirds of paediatric emergencies.

On the subject of the tetanus vaccine, the medical literature mentions, in addition to neurological reactions, acute reactions (anaphylactic shock that can lead to death within hours of vaccination, and especially many respiratory or skin allergies, generalised urticaria, oedema, asthma and others).

In France, we have nothing to envy to the Americans and it is almost more "normal" to be allergic than to live naturally without being forbidden and without risk of allergy.

In France. 10% of school-age children are asthmatic. Young asthmatic children are more sensitive to infections and infections reinforce asthma: they are in a vicious circle as soon as vaccinations are started.

"One child in ten has bronchiolitis (which occurs very frequently after vaccination) and, of those, one in two will develop asthma" (Professor Alain Grimfeld, Tempo Médical, 10 June 1993).

"Young adults who had measles in childhood do not have allergies, unlike those who have been vaccinated and have not had measles." *(*British Medical Journal, 1997)

Eczema-type reactions are linked to the preservatives contained in the vaccine (formaldehyde, mercury, phenoxyethanol, etc.), contaminants from the culture media, antibiotics or disinfectants used during manufacture.

Urticarial reactions are due to the vaccine products themselves or to contaminants such as egg proteins, yeasts, etc.

The number of allergic phenomena seems to obey an exponential law according to the number of doses received, each dose seeming to increase the chronic allergy.

The immune adjuvant - used to increase the immune response - is aluminium hydroxide. This is a chemical that often causes severe allergies and even lesions similar to those seen in BSE (mad cow disease).

In March 2012, MEPs called for a moratorium on aluminium-based vaccines in the name of the precautionary principle. But in June 2012, the Academy of Medicine opposed it, arguing that this adjuvant is necessary for the effectiveness of certain vaccines and that the quantity contained in the injections is much smaller than that which we ingest without noticing it, via water or food.

And for several years now, aluminium has been implicated in Alzheimer's disease.

The Nobel Prize for Medicine and Physiology was awarded in 2006 to two American researchers for their work on interference from "double-stranded RNA" which, in some people, blocks certain genes on the DNA chain. However, among the flu vaccines in general, most contain double RNAs, with the exception of Agrippal, Fluvirine, Gripguard, Influvac and MHG.

This leads Dr Marie-Hélène Groussac, a molecular biology researcher, to say: ***"The flu vaccine is made up of fragments of double-stranded RNA, and therefore blocks certain genes.*** *Injected into elderly people, whose cell genes slow down or reduce their production, it will therefore block certain genes that are already deficient, as explained by the Nobel Prize winner.* ***The result is an abnormal functioning of the cells, in the foreground of which are the neurons!*** *Hence the current growing flowering of Alzheimer's cases, which are putting a strain on the budget and the lives of citizens and which we tend to believe to be inevitable and a source of employment!"*

Aluminium toxicity has been suspected for over twenty years, but has been officially recognised since 1999.

According to the National Health Survey conducted annually by the National Center for Health Statistics, **31% of American children today have a chronic health problem,** 18% require special medical care, and 6.7% have a significant chronic physical or mental disability, of which respiratory allergies, asthma and learning disabilities are the most common.

It is clear that the increasing number of vaccines, given at increasingly early ages to infants, is playing a major role in the increase in all kinds of allergies - the most common chronic childhood illness.

For its part, the Canada Health Survey reported in 1978 that 2.3% of people over the age of 16 years had asthma. By 1991, this figure had risen to 6%. Currently, more than 1.5 million Canadians of all ages suffer from asthma.

In these countries, the percentage of vaccination against hepatitis B, MMR, polio and DTP is 95%.

And in a study comparing 243 vaccinated children to 203 unvaccinated children, Dr. Michel Odent, the famous American pediatrician, reported a high frequency of all diseases, especially ear infections and asthma attacks, among vaccinated children.

After having suggested comparing the health of a group of vaccinated children with that of a corresponding group of unvaccinated children, a study that has never been done in America - nor in France - Dr Philip Incao, an American paediatrician often cited as an expert in trials related to vaccinations, confirmed :

"For 23 years I have observed that unvaccinated children are healthier and stronger than vaccinated children. Allergies, asthma and behavioural disturbances were clearly more common in my young vaccinated patients. On the other hand, they did not suffer more often or more severely from infectious diseases than the others".

He pointed out that the health of children in his country has deteriorated significantly since 1960 with the widespread use of vaccines. Chronic diseases have almost quadrupled since then.

Numerous studies show that by over-stimulating the production of antibodies, vaccinations cause our immune system to panic, which can lead to various reactions such as asthma or allergies.

The response of conventional medicine is to prescribe antihistamines, cortisone and immunosuppressants. All these products, although they provide instant relief, do not cure because they do not act on the cause and also cause significant side effects.

Desensitisation, on the other hand, is not conclusive: it often has the effect of creating new allergies.

Any allergy is caused by an internal disorder; it is the result of an over-reaction of an organism in a state of adaptive incapacity, leading to an inadequate immune response.

It is therefore necessary to restore the vitality of the organism, to strengthen the ground instead of fighting an enemy that is not an enemy. It should be noted that breastfeeding offers good protection against allergies.

Vaccines render the defence system inoperative: overwhelmed by incessant and aggressive antigenic stimulation, it no longer knows how to "cope". So busy fighting its toxic load, our organism allows inflammation to take hold, often for a long time.

The production of antibodies is unbridled, the regulatory mechanisms are overwhelmed, no longer able to carry out their control and cleansing. The permanence of this mass of antibodies produced by repeated vaccinations eventually stops the machine, causing in particular diseases known as **"immune complex diseases".**

In vaccinology, the only objective sought is the production of antibodies: a high level of antibodies is proof, according to the proponents of the vaccine religion, that the vaccine is "effective".

Nothing could be further from the truth. Firstly, antibodies are only a tiny part of the immune processes. Secondly, antibodies are not malleable and can be easily corrupted; **they can cause the exact opposite of an immunisation** and bring about the disease they are supposed to fight, or they can attack our own cells, especially in autoimmune diseases.

All this does not prevent Dr. Jean Pouillard from writing in the Bulletin de l'ordre des médecins of 20 December 2003: *"... a recent article shows that, during their first five years, children with high vaccination coverage seem to be even better protected than others against the development of allergies."*

Autism

Dr Andrew Wakefield, a gastroenterologist and director of a research group at the Royal Free Hospital, London School of Medicine, is an international authority on drug-induced intestinal diseases.

He and his team have been working for years on the causal links between the measles virus in the MMR vaccine, autism and intestinal disorders in children.

It should be noted that today there is 1 case in 500 children, and there are even 40 suspected cases per 10,000, or 1 case in 250.

It has been discovered that the weakening of the immune system is actually a syndrome in autistic people.

Specialists in allergy, immunology, neurology and biochemistry have noted that autism is becoming more and more widespread and there is now enough evidence to suggest that autism should be considered as a neuroimmunological disorder..:

It is therefore becoming increasingly clear that regressive autism should be associated with the measles, mumps and rubella (MMR) vaccine.

Autism does appear to be an autoimmune disease of vaccine origin.

Autism increased thirty-fold between 1978 and 1999 in the United States and London. This corresponds to the vaccination

campaigns (MMR) in these two countries. There is no such thing as chance.

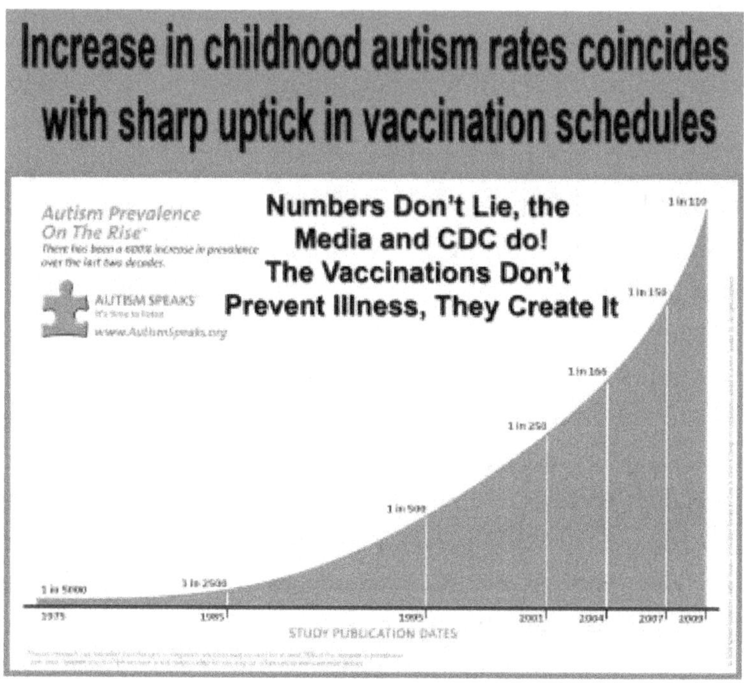

Autism begins, before the age of three, with a delay or total absence of spoken language development, often with repetitive movements. The child presents excessive thirst, intestinal disorders, a tendency to self-mutilation and, very often, an atopic terrain and a fragility of the respiratory tract, which places us in the tuberculinous terrain.

Remember that the three vaccines against measles, mumps and rubella are live, attenuated but live viruses!

Let us also recall that Great Britain and Germany have banned MMR on their territory, after having observed about three hundred cases of meningitis.

France continued its vaccination policy, claiming that there was no problem, that the vaccine was reliable.

In the United States, the Californian health authorities noted a 273% increase in autism cases in 10 years!

In 1965, parents had already noticed the onset of autism in their child after the injection of the triple DTP vaccine. When another triple vaccine was introduced in 1980, MMR, "alarming reports from parents increased dramatically" (Los Angeles Time, April 26, 2000).

The law firm Dawbarns of Norfolk, England, has handled more than 600 cases of complications following the MMR vaccine. Among these complications, the cases, published on June 3, 1997 and regularly updated, report 287 cases of autism.

This autism-vaccine relationship demonstrates to perfection the inability of most doctors, whether specialists or general practitioners, to imagine the possibility of a link between vaccination and post-vaccination accident.

Over the past ten years, many parents reported that their child, who was developing normally, **had begun to show symptoms related to autism soon after receiving the MMR vaccine.**

The stories from the United States, the United Kingdom, Canada and other countries are all similar: a healthy child who had previously passed through all stages of development successfully receives the MMR vaccine. He or she then stops learning new skills and words and then loses ground and eventually regresses to autism.

According to the Center for Disease Control and Prevention and the manufacturers of the vaccine, this is just a coincidence.

In children whose mothers have immune disease, the incidence is nine times higher than in other children.

THE FLU IN FRANCE
KEY FIGURES FOR THE 2014-2015 FLU EPIDEMIC :
- Nearly 2.9 million consultations for flu syndrome
- More than 3,133 hospitalizations reported by emergency services
- 1,558 severe cases of influenza admitted to intensive care units
- 53% were not vaccinated
- Excess of 18,300 deaths from all causes, 90% of which were among the elderly (65 years and over).
- The cost of the 2014-2015 flu epidemic was €180 million.

If 53% were not vaccinated, doesn't that mean that of the 2,900,000 people who caught the flu, 47% were vaccinated, or 1,363,000 people?

The report on the 2009 influenza A "epidemic".

Registered at the Presidency of the National Assembly on 6 July 2010, this report was made on behalf of the commission of enquiry into the way in which the vaccination campaign against influenza A(H1N1) was programmed, explained and managed.

The report consists of 172 pages, of which the following paragraphs are a summary:

A public health failure

The vaccination campaign against the A(H1N1) virus has led to two observations: on the one hand, the objective of mass vaccination of the population is far from being achieved, and on the other hand, there is dissatisfaction on the part of the

health professionals, especially private doctors and nurses, who seem to have moved away from the health authorities for a long time.

A low vaccination rate

According to the information provided by the Director General of the National Health Insurance Fund for Salaried Workers (CNAMTS), Mr Frédéric van Roekeghem, the total number of people vaccinated in France against influenza A(H1N1) could eventually reach 5.7 million. The Department of Health Emergencies similarly estimates vaccination coverage at 5.36 million people on 1 June 2010, i.e. less than 8.5% of the total population.

A lack of understanding between health authorities and health professionals

... Mr. Claude Le Pen, professor of economics at the University of Paris-Dauphine, judged that if a new massive vaccination campaign were to be envisaged, *"the extraordinary potential of the country's 50,000 private doctors, 60,000 nurses, 3,000 hospitals and 22,000 pharmacies would undoubtedly not be excluded from the system. These professionals felt very badly about their exclusion and emitted antibodies more because of this exclusion than because of the health policy itself".*

Many uncertainties

"The flu virus is a misleading and misleading virus": it was with these words that Professor Claude Hannoun, who in 1950 invented France's first flu vaccine, reminded the commission of enquiry of the fundamentally unpredictable nature of the flu, which, sixty years after the first vaccine was developed, remains relatively unknown.

... In any case, the experience of the A(H1N1) flu pandemic remains rich in lessons: it led to an unprecedented mobilization of industrialists, who showed in this crisis context, a great reactivity and a real ability to adapt their production lines.

A vaccination pre-strategy aimed at complete protection of the population

Why has France chosen to order 94 million doses of vaccine? This decision, taken on 3 July 2009 by the Prime Minister, is easy to explain: the question is, however, whether it was justified.

The willingness to conclude other contracts quickly

GlaxoSmithKline said it was prepared to commit to making 50 million doses available to France in deliveries spread over October to December 2009 provided a firm commitment is made before midnight on 12 May. The green light given by the Prime Minister on 11 May led the office of the Minister for Health to send a letter of intent to the laboratory on 14 May to preserve 50 million doses of the future vaccine at a cost of 75 million euros. Production of the Pandemrix vaccine then began on 22 June.

Was it necessary to set a more modest target for vaccine coverage?

According to the opinions of the experts heard by the commission of enquiry, a barrier vaccination strategy implies immunising 30% of the population, which would make it possible to halt the exponential spread of an epidemic or pandemic. However, this model has never been tested in practice: in fact, no country has ever implemented such a vaccination strategy.

Difficulties related to the operating rules of the centres

The planned rhythm of injections also seemed incompatible with normal exercise: it was in fact planned that, at full speed, the centres would allow one person to be vaccinated every two minutes; the nursing staff strongly criticised this objective, even going so far as to compare it to "veterinary medicine".

A multiplicity of confusing health messages

Thus, on 6 May 2009, Professor Antoine Flahault, Director of the École des hautes études en santé publique, gave an interview to the newspaper Le Monde in which he evoked several scenarios for the possible evolution of the disease; according to him, the most plausible scenario was close to the 1968 pandemic, namely "the equivalent of a major seasonal flu affecting 35% of the population, with "an excess of mortality in the order of 20,000 to 30,000 deaths in France", numbers that are necessarily impressive. However, on 28 August 2009, Professor François Bricaire, head of the infectious and tropical diseases department at the Pitié-Salpêtrière, told the Figaro Magazine: *"This flu is mostly benign."*

The reluctance of care workers

... The evocation of a "grippette" had, as we remember, an effect, if not devastating, at least a very clear impact. We will also recall the positions taken in October 2009, in the Parisien, by Mr Patrick Pelloux, president of the Association of hospital emergency doctors, who declared: *"I don't see the scientific interest of this vaccine",* and *Professor David Khayat, head of the cancerology department of the Pitié-Salpêtrière hospital, who announced: "No, I won't be vaccinated (...). I am waiting for the arguments that would justify such a mass vaccination."*

Worrying messages about vaccine safety

... A widely publicised controversy has arisen over the safety of pandemic vaccines, based on misunderstandings and confusion, which has led to the use of adjuvants being called into question, while at the same time raising concerns about the possible risk of Guillain-Barré syndrome. France was one of the countries where the main argument against vaccination was the risk incurred by vaccines considered insufficiently safe.

The debate on adjuvants also received a lot of media attention: the vaccines were said to contain substances whose dangerousness was not well known, since pregnant women and children aged between six and twenty-four months with risk factors - which was in fact a precautionary measure linked to the very particular nature of their immune systems - were not daring to give them.

As for Guillain-Barré syndrome, which had hitherto been little known to the public, it too was able to experience its media "hour of glory", especially since the first case, observed in a vaccinated healthcare worker, was made public on 12 November 2009, the date of the launch of the campaign targeting the general population.

The need for a public debate on the risks of a pandemic or serious health crisis

... In addition, it would no doubt be appropriate to organise, as was the case for bioethics, a general meeting on the challenges of vaccination in general, which would enable a panel of citizens representative of the population, previously trained in the issue, to conduct a debate informed by scientists on vaccination policy in France.

Finally, we need to conduct a proactive public information campaign to remind the general public of the benefits of vaccination and to fight against vaccination refusal and, more widely, to spread a public health culture, particularly among the most disadvantaged groups, so that we can mobilise our fellow citizens during the next health crisis.

What you need to know about this report

- The change in the definition of the pandemic by the MMR on 5 June 2009 is at the origin of the gigantic orders for vaccines by the different States of the planet.

- The AH1N1 influenza vaccine would never have received a marketing authorisation.

- Parliamentarians would only have had 24 hours to go and consult the text on the spot without even the right to photocopy it to study it at leisure.

- While there had never been a double vaccination in the case of a flu, the WHO recommended it for the AH1N1 flu.

Moreover, the organisation of a general meeting on the issues of vaccination would indeed be an excellent thing. But how do they intend to organise them? What do the terms "previously trained on the issue" mean in terms of the citizens who would take part in them?

Shouldn't "conformed" be read rather than "trained"? As for the "debate informed by scientists", since they would have to "remind people of the benefits of vaccination and fight against vaccination refusal", it is quite obvious that the opponents of vaccination, those irresponsible, paranoid people, would not be invited to it!

Move along, there's nothing to see... and nothing to say!

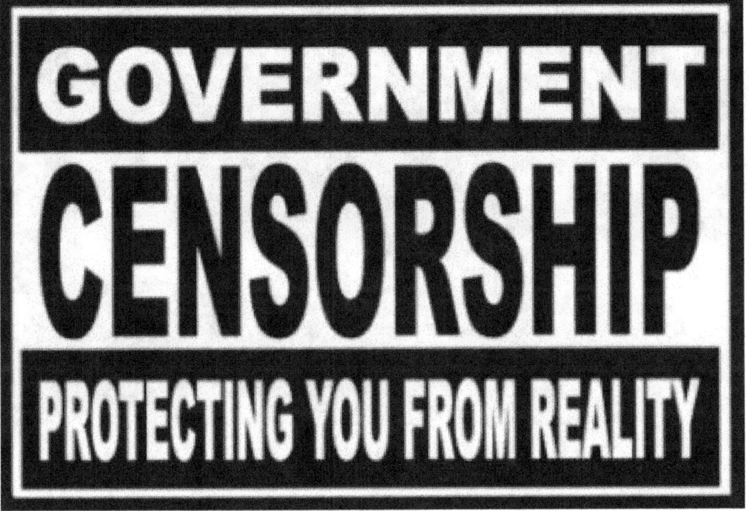

But still

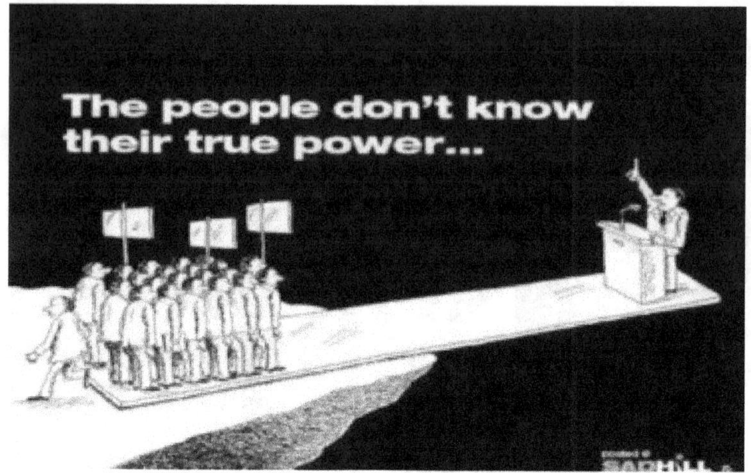

THE COST OF THE 2009 AH1N1 INFLUENZA

The Budget Minister at the time had announced, before the National Assembly, that expenditure on influenza A would amount to 1.5 billion euros. But the Senate's finance committee had instead estimated the cost at 1.8 to 2 billion euros, distributed in this way:

- Purchase of 94 million doses = 1.5 billion €

- Vaccination campaign = 35.8 million €

- Purchase of antivirals = 20 million €

- Purchase of masks = 150.6 million €

- Logistical expenses = 41.6 million €

- Compensation for personnel requisitioned
= 290 million €

- Information costs = 59.6 million €

- Costs related to territorial organisation
of the campaign = 100 million €

- Expenditure related to doctor's consultations, prescription of medicines, sick leave = 375 to 752 million €

In the end, only 5.3 million vaccines were used, which is a good thing, but it means that several million doses went into the trash once the expiry date was reached.

The parliamentary report estimates the cost of the fiasco at 668.35 million €. It feels a bit like the day after a demonstration when the interior ministry and the participants give their respective figures.

BABY VACCINE OR BABY SHAKE?

In the United States, Alan Yurko spent several years of his life in prison for the murder of his child, accused of mistreating him. The reason? No sooner had his 10-week-old child been vaccinated than he died shortly afterwards. The child also showed characteristic petechiae (small red to purplish spots on the skin) and signs of fractures.

Alan Yurko was sentenced to life imprisonment and was eventually released after 6 years of detention thanks to a reopening of his case and further analysis by independent doctors.

The vaccine had caused the same damage to his child's brain, found at autopsy, as would have been caused if he had mistreated his child.

Petechiae are a haemorrhagic phenomenon, but hexavalent vaccines (such as Infanrix hexa for example), have already been associated by forensic doctors with phenomena of fatal cerebral oedemas in infants.

THE ZIKA VIRUS, THE NEW FEAR

At an emergency meeting on 1 February 2016, the World Health Organisation announced that the Zika virus, inoculated by the tiger mosquito, could affect 3 to 4 million people worldwide. The W.H.O. also decreed that the epidemic constitutes "a public health emergency of global concern" by declaring a red alert, the fourth in its history.

The Zika virus disease is however relatively benign and does not require any specific treatment, as researcher Elias Zehrouni pointed out:

*"For the vast majority of cases, Zika is **a mild infection…** One person in five shows symptoms. The real problem is the pregnant woman. How can we succeed in protecting pregnant women or women of childbearing age?"*

On this subject, the W.M.S. states: *"The health authorities are currently investigating the possible link between the Zika virus disease in pregnant women and microcephaly in newborn babies". Officially, no causality has been established between Zika and the cerebral malformation in the infant, but it is strongly suspected."*

But is it really this virus that causes developmental delays in the foetuses of infected pregnant women, resulting in microcephalies? Are we on the trail of the real culprit? The Brazilian association for collective health Abrasco and the Argentinean organisation PCST "Physicians in the Crop-Sprayed Towns" point to a completely different culprit: pyriproxyfen.

This larvicide, developed by the Japanese company Sumitomo Chemical, a partner of Monsanto, has been injected since the end of 2014 into collective rainwater reservoirs intended for consumption by the inhabitants of the north-eastern part of the country.

Pyriproxyfen is a growth inhibitor and effectively prevents the development of mosquito larvae. However, Abrasco doctors draw a direct parallel between the symptoms this insecticide causes in mosquitoes and the malformations of newborns in areas where drinking water has been treated. They also point out that north-eastern Brazil is the only region to experience such an outbreak of microcephalus cases. According to their figures, there are 30 times more cases than in the north and at least 300 times more than in the south.

At the time of writing, the origin of the disease is not certain for the tiger mosquito or for pyriproxyfen. On the other hand, if **it is indeed the pesticide which is the cause of the microcephalies** and that it is not recognised as such, we would be in a typical case of a vicious circle since by pouring the pesticide intended to exterminate the innocent mosquito we would cause the malformations of the infants!

Still, Sanofi laboratories have announced that they are launching into the race for the vaccine, specifying on February 9, 2016 that they will launch a clinical trial in one year's time. The British giant GSK, the main competitor, has announced that it is undertaking feasibility studies.

In India, the Bharat Biotech laboratory announced that two vaccines against this virus had been in gestation for a year and were now ready to be tested on animals. *"We are the first in the world to apply for a licence for a vaccine against the Zika virus,"* said Rajarshi Dasgupta, head of the laboratory's intellectual property department, adding that the application for a licence had been made a year ago.

In the United States, U.S. President Barack Obama announced his intention to release 1.8 billion dollars for prevention and research on Zika.

In mainland France, the Institut de veille sanitaire (Health Watch Institute) has sent the first report on the number of travellers who contracted Zika in an affected area and returned to mainland France: 5 people have shown symptoms since the beginning of 2016. None of the patients presented any serious form of infection.

Questions and Answers

Assuming that a link has been proven between Zika virus disease in pregnant women and microcephaly in newborn babies, once they have issued their vaccine, will the laboratories be content to vaccinate only the 800,000 pregnant women in France each year or will they try, as with the papillomavirus, to vaccinate all teenage girls?

And what will it be like in Brazil (1.5 million recorded cases) where the population is 204 million and the birth rate 15%?

And what about the world's population of 1.2 billion adolescents aged 10 to 19, or about 500 million young girls?

The future will tell us...

In France, the VACCINAL OBLIGATION IS OUTSIDE THE LAW.

- ANTICONSTITUTIONAL: Article 3 of the Universal Declaration of Human Rights: *"Everyone has the right to life, liberty and security of person."*

- CONTREDITED BY THE CIVIL CODE Article 16-3. *"The integrity of the human body may only be damaged in cases of therapeutic necessity for the person. The consent of the person concerned must be obtained beforehand, except in cases where his or her condition necessitates a therapeutic intervention to which he or she is not in a position to consent."*

- CONTRARY TO THE MEDICAL DEONTOLOGY CODE: Article 36 (Article R.4127-36 of the Public Health Code). *"The consent of the person being examined or treated must be sought in all cases. When the patient, in a state of being able to express his will, refuses the proposed investigations or treatment, the doctor must respect this refusal after having informed the patient of the consequences. If the patient is unable to express his or her wishes, the doctor may not intervene without informing the patient's family and friends, unless it is urgent or impossible to do so. The physician's obligations towards the patient when the patient is a minor or a protected adult are defined in Article 42."*

Article L.1111-4 of the Public Health Code specifies in this respect: *"Any person shall take, with the health professional and taking into account the information and recommendations provided by him, decisions concerning his health. The doctor must respect the will of the person after having informed him/her of the consequences of his/her choices. If the person's willingness to refuse or interrupt any treatment is life-threatening, the doctor must do everything possible to convince the person to accept the necessary treatment. He or she may call on another member of the medical profession. In all cases, the patient must reiterate his or her decision after a reasonable period of time. The decision is recorded in the patient's medical file. The doctor safeguards the dignity of the dying person and ensures the quality of his or her end-of-life by providing the care referred to in Article L. 1110-10."*

- Contrary to the Court judgments of 25 FEBRUARY and 14 OCTOBER 1997: *"Information to patients: practitioners must be able to prove that they have provided the patient with fair, clear, appropriate and exhaustive information, at least on the slightest risks. The purpose of this information is to enable the patient to refuse the proposed vaccination on the grounds that the risks outweigh the expected benefits".*

- CONTRARY TO THE EUROPEAN CONVENTION ON HUMAN RIGHTS: On 9 July 2002, the European Court of Human Rights ruled in a decision concerning an Italian national that compulsory vaccination, as involuntary medical treatment, constituted an interference with the right to respect for private and family life guaranteed by Article 8 of the European Convention.

- CONTRARY TO THE LAW OF 4 MARCH 2002 - No. 2002-303, Article 11, Chapter 1, amending Art. L 1111-4 of Chapter 1 of Title 1 of Book 1 of Part 1 of the Public Health Code: *"No medical act or treatment may be practised without the free and informed consent of the person, and such consent may be withdrawn at any time".*

- Contrary to the Convention on the Rights of the Child (1989)

- Contrary to the Oviedo Convention on Human Rights and Biomedicine (1997)

- Contrary to the European Convention on Patients' Rights (2002)

- Contrary to the International Covenant on Civil and Political Rights (1966)

- Contrary to the Nuremberg Code (a set of ethical principles on research in the field of medical experimentation established in 1947 after the Nuremberg Trial at the end of the Second World War).

A CHILD'S IMMUNE SYSTEM IS NOT FINISHED BEFORE THE AGE OF 3!

Ignoring or denying this fact is equivalent, no more and no less, to thinking like the 16th century obscurantists who condemned Galileo!

Whose idea was it to make a baby drink a large glass of whisky or vodka just out of its mother's womb? And how else would such an act be qualified as criminal?

Injecting live, attenuated or dead viruses into an organism that is in no state to defend itself is just as absurd. It is to consider the marvel that is the human body as an unfinished machine, as if nature had not provided it with everything it needs to stay healthy.

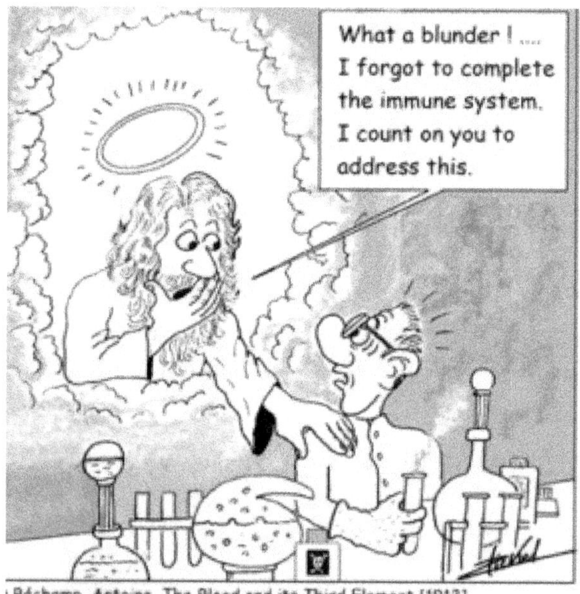

Béchamp, Antoine, The Blood and its Third Element [1912]

Among the little victims, it is the babies of the so-called "emerging" countries such as India who pay the heaviest price for the vaccine octopus, since manufacturers of powdered milk encourage mothers not to breastfeed their children in favour of their products. And what water do they put in their bottles?

These unfortunate children are therefore being inflicted with this explosive cocktail: absence of breast milk + bottles filled with non-potable water + diphtheria, tetanus, polio, hepatitis B, measles etc. vaccines !

Are their lives less valuable than ours?

The cherry tree gives its fruit at the beginning of summer and loses its leaves in autumn, that's how it is. The sun rises in the morning, sets in the evening and does not revolve around the earth, that's how it is. The immune system builds and strengthens itself during the first three years of life, that's how it works.

These are the laws of nature where needle trees do not exist. To go against nature is to play sorcerer's apprentice, which has been done for 150 years.

Laura Hayes speaks on the "Age of Autism" website

"I think it's critically important for everyone to understand that the term 'safe vaccines' is an oxymoron, and therefore I would say that even those who claim to be 'pro-science' would not be able to agree that there is an 'intelligent approach to vaccination' if they were properly and fully informed. By their very nature, vaccines cannot be made safe, because they artificially stimulate the immune system in an unnatural way (direct injection of toxic cocktails into the body, whereas nature provides other "doors": inhalation or ingestion. This is how the first part of the immune response is bypassed, whereas this part is essential to ensure the correct subsequent responses .

It is a bit like intervening during a woman's pregnancy, forcing the order of things, eliminating certain critical stages, while thinking that this way of doing things will not have an impact on the final result). This is how dangerous adjuvants (such as neurotoxic aluminium, or proteins) cannot be degraded in the circulatory system, whereas these processes must take place in the gastrointestinal tract. The same also applies to neurotoxins such as mercury and aluminium, which are injected at a period of child development when the blood-brain barrier is wide open. All this is foreign to the functioning of the immune system. It can be concluded that "safe vaccines" are a first-rate oxymoron. If you then multiply these dangerous procedures by administering several vaccines at the same time, without taking into account family data, the weight of the child, without making sure that there are no allergies and metabolic problems, then you have the recipe for a possible absolute disaster.

Therefore, since there are no "safe vaccines", we inevitably end up having to discuss freedom of medical choice, which must ALWAYS be an essential component in any free and ethical society. This is all the more important, however, because vaccine manufacturers, like those who administer them, are relieved of all responsibility thanks to the incredible "National Childhood Vaccine Injury Act" of 1986 (you only have to look at the actual wording of this Act to realise that "safe vaccines" is an oxymoron). In 1986, at a time when the number of vaccines should have been reduced (I would like to say that they should have been stopped altogether) following all the damage and deaths caused by these vaccines, following all the complaints and lawsuits that followed, vaccinations were paradoxically increased and even tripled *once compensation and indemnification was put in place. Let's talk about something CLEAR!*

Today, vaccine exemptions are limited, under attack and in danger of disappearing throughout the country. All this must stop and freedom of medical choice must be protected and enforced in all 50 states for all medical procedures and treatments, including vaccinations. A scientific and intelligent approach to vaccination must always include the option of being able to say NO, without government interference, coercion, or any cost whatsoever.

Informed consent, which implies the possibility to say freely YES or NO without any constraint, is closely linked to the freedom of medical choice and must therefore ALWAYS be an essential component of any free society where fundamental ethics are respected. As far as vaccines are concerned, this is unfortunately not possible because they have never been properly studied, either individually or in the countless combinations with which they are administered, or even globally during the first 18 years of a child's life.

So any information that a doctor can give on the benefits of vaccines is not only not complete and factual information, but can only be strictly personal information....which is not based on any solid science. This is especially true when doctors and the government proclaim that there is no link between vaccines and autism, given what we now know about Dr. Paul Thorsen. Many people base their opinions on this doctor's studies to say that there is no link between vaccines and autism. It is important to remember that this man stole money from the US government to do a study on the relationship between vaccines and autism. While this man is wanted as a fugitive, it is his worthless study that is constantly being relied upon. Let's talk about FOLIE again! It must be said once again that "true science, an intelligent approach to vaccination" must always give way to free and informed consent, which obviously includes the right to accept or refuse some or even all vaccines without any interference, constraint or cost.

In the case of vaccines, informed consent is also compromised because our own government agencies have been bent on hiding uncomfortable truths for decades now. This cover-up includes the fact that the toxic amounts of thiomersal that were in vaccines from the 1980s to the early 2000s were statistically and closely linked to autism, not to mention a whole series of debilitating childhood epidemics that we have witnessed in this country. For those who are not aware of what I am talking about, all they need to do is Google search for "Verstraeten", "Simpsonwood" and "Brick Township, NJ".

In addition, there can be no informed consent because the companies that manufacture and profit from the sale of the vaccines are doing the studies. Unlike an independent regulatory body that could afford to lose billions if the tests performed did not reflect what they had hoped for. Isn't that a bit like the fox guarding the henhouse? You can't trust any study that comes from the industry. These studies are misleading and worthless. They are short-term studies that test a new vaccine against another vaccine or against a dangerous and highly reactive adjuvant like aluminum, instead of a neutral saline solution. This is the problem of fake placebo. It is a bit like saying that cocaine (crack) is safe and non-addictive, because it is no more dangerous than heroin! The kind of studies that pharmaceutical companies have presented as valid are in fact fraudulent, and these companies should be charged with criminal negligence and worse.

Finally, there are no adequate data to reflect the incredible number of adverse vaccine reactions, including vaccine-induced deaths. This is because our VAERS (Vaccine Adverse Events Reporting System) is a passive and voluntary system. I find this almost impossible to believe, but it is a fact. Not only are doctors not required to report vaccine damage and deaths to this system (VAERS), but most of them don't even know it exists! Until such reporting becomes mandatory, until doctors are actually trained to examine vaccine damage and follow up, for at least one year, all patients who have been vaccinated, until severe penalties (including permanent loss of their licence) can be imposed on doctors who fail to report vaccine side effects, no one, absolutely no one, will be able to know the extent and nature of the devastating effects of the national vaccination programme. Unfortunately, we do not have this data because those in power, and those who profit from the situation, do not want the public to have access to this information.

I think that the community of individuals and families who have suffered vaccine damage or the parents of people who have died after vaccines must continue to shed light on all the issues that have been raised in this article. I think that vaccination is a barbaric practice that is not based on any science worthy of the name. We now have a mountain of evidence that shows us that these practices should stop immediately.

O.M.S. EVALUATION REPORT 2014 THE GLOBAL ACTION PLAN FOR VACCINES

Strategic Advisory Group experts on vaccination

The Global Vaccine Action Plan (GVAP) has two main ambitions :

First, universal immunization: 1.5 million children still die each year from diseases that can be prevented by the vaccines humanity has developed.

Second, to unleash the vast future potential of vaccines: Their impressive history to date is only the foundation for the great successes of the future.

... With these two great ambitions, the Global Action Plan for Vaccines aims to make the decade 2011-2020 the "Decade of Immunization" ...

The Action Plan sets six key targets for immunization with target dates at the end of 2014 or 2015. Only one of these targets is on track to be achieved .

... There is, however, reason for hope. The introduction of new vaccines has had some success, and positive changes have occurred in some countries. A major change is possible. The Global Action Plan for Vaccines was created to end global inequities in immunization and thereby save millions of lives .

... This imperative remains as important and urgent as ever. It is unacceptable that the Plan fails to achieve results on the scale required....

... Basic flaws in integration mean that health workers repeatedly miss easy opportunities to offer vaccinations when patients come for other problems...

To put it plainly: when a patient comes in for a cold or headache, take the opportunity to offer vaccinations. Healthcare workers must therefore be better trained in marketing, following the example of their master in this field: Louis Pasteur.

... The distribution of vaccines faces difficult situations, such as wars or major outbreaks of disease (such as Ebola at present). There will always be such situations, but the vaccines must still be distributed...

Let the countries at war tell themselves: even under the bombs, it is necessary to vaccinate!

... The global action plan for vaccines is vital. Vaccines are remarkable products. They protect against diseases that can scar, kill and maim.

... It is estimated that they prevent 2 to 3 million deaths per year. They are the ones we look for when a new disease emerges. Compared to their great benefits, their cost is reduced.

... Vaccines: an impressive history and an exciting future ... Widespread vaccination was one of the great public health revolutions of the 20th century and the future is even more promising...

Promising for whom?

... By keeping deadly or crippling communicable diseases under control, vaccines are, and will remain, essential for maintaining and developing health gains... They can "make a difference" in the face of future outbreaks and epidemics...

... Vaccines are already preventing certain cancers caused by viruses and, increasingly, they will prevent non-communicable diseases and will have a beneficial effect at any age...

Soon cancer vaccines for children and infants?

... Vaccines have an exciting future, but the need is greatest in the present.

Exhilarating future for whom?

This report provides an objective assessment of progress. It is written by the Decade of Immunization working group within the Strategic Advisory Group of Experts on Immunization (SAGE), based on analyses and deliberations throughout the year.

Immunization for All: Progress is lagging far behind. The Global Action Plan for Vaccines envisioned a world in which every person could enjoy a life free of vaccine-preventable diseases. It aims to extend the full benefits of immunization to all people, wherever they are born, wherever they live and whoever they may be. In all cases, it is about improving the coverage and reliability of immunization services so that children who are not yet properly immunized can be reached.

The Indians of the Amazon or the Australian Bush just have to behave themselves...

Preparedness for global epidemics and emergencies :

Countries at risk of epidemics need preparedness plans that are firmly anchored in their overall immunization plans and services.

Similarly, there is a need to be able to respond quickly and appropriately to emergencies and natural disasters at national and global levels, as the response may involve the rational use of vaccines.

With respect to influenza, a global network of laboratories is monitoring circulating virus strains and all countries need up-to-date pandemic preparedness plans.

In many cases, however, preparedness plans are too old, unworkable or simply non-existent. Governments, WHO, UNICEF, vaccine manufacturers and research institutes are currently supporting the development of national preparedness plans and are working to develop the potential for global influenza vaccine production, including work to develop a new vaccine against virus strains with pandemic potential.

It should be noted that 45% of Unicef's funds are earmarked for immunization in Third World countries, while only 17% are devoted to water and sanitation, even though a report by Unicef states that "one person in five in the world still does not have access to water and a reliable water supply system"!

Children in the Third World need clean water and food, not aggressive agents that kill them like flies. Massive vaccinations in African countries have decimated these populations but we still persist in vaccinating!

Better still, the world authorities have launched the V.E.P. (Expanded Programme on Universal Childhood Immunization) whose objective is the vaccination of all the children of the world against the six most common diseases of early childhood: poliomyelitis, diphtheria, tetanus, measles, whooping cough, tuberculosis.

How dare to say that diphtheria, tetanus and poliomyelitis are common diseases of early childhood?

Some equally terrifying notes from the World Health Organization.

- Vaccination against Hepatitis B:

Since early perinatal or postnatal transmission is a major cause of chronic infections worldwide, the first dose should be given as soon as possible (within 24 hours) after birth, even in low endemic countries.

The first vaccination against hepatitis B usually consists of 3 doses of vaccine (i.e. 1 dose of monovalent vaccine at birth, followed by 2 doses of monovalent or combined vaccine). However, for programmatic reasons, 4 doses may be given (e.g., 1 dose of monovalent vaccine at birth, followed by 3 doses of monovalent or combined vaccine), according to the schedules of national routine immunization programmes.

Some infants born prematurely with low birth weight (2000 g) may not respond well to vaccination at birth. However, at the chronological age of one month, these preterm infants are likely to show a sufficient response regardless of their birth weight or initial gestational age. Therefore, doses given to children weighing less than 2000g should not be counted as part of the primary vaccination series...

- Vaccination against Poliomyelitis :

Zero dose OPV should be given at birth or as soon as possible thereafter to maximize seroconversion rates and induce mucosal protection.

Administration of the primary series, consisting of 3 doses of OPV plus 1 dose of IPV, may begin at 6 weeks of age, with a minimum interval of 4 weeks between OPV doses. If a single dose of IPV is used, it should be given from 14 weeks of age (when maternal antibodies have declined and immunogenicity is significantly increased) and may be given at the same time as OPV.

For infants starting late in the routine immunization schedule (at less than 3 months of age), the dose of IPV should be given at the first immunization contact.

- Vaccination against Tetanus :

A tetanus vaccination schedule of 5 doses is recommended during childhood. Ideally, a booster should be given between 4 and 7 years of age, followed by another booster during adolescence, for example between 12 and 15 years of age. Tetanus booster doses can use DTP or Td depending on the age of the child. The Td vaccine should be used for Tetanus booster doses and Diphtheria beyond age 7.

Interview with Dr Françoise Berthoud, paediatrician, homeopathic doctor

Journalist: *Can you tell us about the health of the unvaccinated children in your clientele?*

Françoise Berthoud: *I'm currently retired but I worked in Geneva in Switzerland and it's true that, in any case among the children I had from when I was very young or even from the mother's womb, and especially among those who chose not to have any vaccinations at all, it's remarkable the health of these children who we never actually see and who don't have the chronic ear infections and bronchitis of all their little friends in the building.*

So it's a subject I've studied a lot, well already the popular wisdom, all the mothers who have told me: the children of the neighbours who have all been vaccinated are always sick, mine never.

Someone who says to me: my 16 year old daughter, she has never had any vaccinations, when she is sick it lasts 3 days, things like that. That's the daily life of this type of medicine.

I also looked in the literature what I found, and all around the world there are people who have done studies, especially with children who have not received the pertussis vaccine.

This has been done by Michel Audan on the one hand, who is a French obstetrician surgeon who is now in London and who is studying the consequences of very young age on the pathology of the adolescent or adult in an institute.

He has taken children either from the Steiner school or from extended breastfeeding groups who had not been vaccinated against whooping cough and he has statistically proven that these children had up to 4 times less asthma in their childhood.

There is also something very interesting, and that is in relation to autism, there are many, many studies that are being done, not by conventional doctors but by other people on the relationship between autism and vaccination.

On the one hand the role of mercury, heavy metals in vaccines, and on the other hand the role of the measles vaccine virus. Autism is a behavioural problem which is 300 times more frequent now than when it was first described some 50 years ago and many researchers attribute this to vaccinations and other pollution such as dental amalgams etc.

And it has been proved that there is no autism and also much less asthma in two important communities in the United States, on the one hand the Amish community who are people who live in the countryside with rites that date back several centuries, and in another community in Chicago where doctors give birth at home called Home-First and follow tens of thousands of children with very little or no vaccinations.

Journalist: *Can you tell us about what is called homeopathic vaccination drainage?*

Françoise Berthoud: *Yes, that's a very interesting subject: some homeopaths actually drain or clean vaccines with medicines, it may be a good thing but that's not what I've learned, what I've learned is what is called isopathic drainage, that is to say that we take the very substance of the vaccine and make it into a homeopathic medicine by dilution-dynamisation.*

And I have to say that I have some very nice stories in my daily life as a homeopathic pediatrician about that. I remember in particular one day when I spoke on television about the measles, mumps, rubella vaccine and the doubts about this vaccination.

I had had two or three phone calls, one of which was from a mother who said to me: listen, I don't know if you can do anything because since this vaccination my child is out, he no longer has any joie de vivre.

I told him, well come and see me, I had time to see him quite quickly, and I remember very, very well this child who was 15 or 18 months old and who was on his mother's lap and who was completely asleep. His mother was saying: yes, he has no life anymore, in fact.

Every week I gave him what I usually gave him: isopathic vaccine and I made this lady come back. It wasn't my habit to make people come back, I told them: no news, good news, but now I really wanted to see.

And I saw a little child completely transformed, absolutely alive, starting to make noise as soon as he entered the waiting room. And the mother said to me: it was fascinating, with each dose he woke up like a flower that you water!

And there are lots of other stories like that. Well, that doesn't mean it always works, it doesn't mean: go ahead and vaccinate happily, we'll be able to drain you without any problem. To vaccinate, not to vaccinate, it's a huge subject.

As a practitioner, what I was trying to look for was what was right for that family. There are families for whom it is right not to vaccinate at all, there are others who still have fears like tetanus.

So when I did vaccinations, I always followed up with drainage, even when there were no symptoms. Or if people came with an older child who had been to other doctors before, who had been vaccinated and received antibiotics etc., I would do a drainage treatment of everything he had received.

Conference by Doctor Didier Tarte on 29 November 2013 at the Palais des Congrès in Namur

I was trained like all my colleagues on the model of the single thought... afterwards, gradually, I met people who woke me up, patients in particular and I was lucky enough to meet the League for Vaccination Freedom in 1987 which gave me the means to understand what was happening.

The league was connected to a central office that sent them all the documents, articles and publications that evoked the word vaccine... and there I had the proof that there were a lot of problems around vaccines, a lot of publications that showed the side effects that did not then appear in the official press because the laboratories had all the medical and scientific press.

I was an occupational physician for the last 13 years of my activity, which I finished in 2011, and there I was able to touch the way the system worked.

I was threatened several times by the Council of the Order, which implied that, in the end, I risked being sanctioned and disbarred.

At the end of my activity they tried to have my skin anyway and they asked me to go before their assembly because I had very often mentioned in my activity the problems posed by vaccinations because I was horrified by what I saw in my practice as an occupational physician.

And I refrained from going to see them because they are people who have no respect, no attention to others and so I resigned.

What I found: the muscular suffering of people is terrible. So I started to look through the health records, I saw a multiplication of aberrant vaccines, people were being over-vaccinated against tetanus every 5 years - according to the law it was every 10 years but it was no problem for the doctors to multiply the vaccines.

And when the hepatitis B vaccine arrived, in 1994 in a generalised manner, and that was spread enormously among adolescents, because in the strategy of the laboratories they had already created a consortium with the WHO to prepare the ground: to make the WHO aware of the problem of hepatitis... they thought about the strategy to put in place and they knew that there was a part of the population that was resistant to health action.

Who was it? It was the teenagers. So they set up a strategy: if we can get the teenagers, we'll get the population. So everything was based, to get the teenagers to fall for it, through the kiss that was supposed to transmit the hepatitis virus... Great hype with the help of all the media and we generalised the vaccination against hepatitis B to the point that, having had the teenagers, half of the French were vaccinated against Hepatitis B.

To validate my activity as an occupational physician, I was asked to write a dissertation during my training... I wrote a dissertation where I simply wondered... because I followed 57 garbage collectors in a Community of Communes that I took charge of in 2001 and in 2003 I wrote a dissertation in the following direction.

I had noticed that these people had very poor health, many accidents at work, a lot of work stoppages, some for almost a year... I made an exhaustive list of all the vaccinations received by each person and I identified the 10 people who had received the most vaccinations and the 10 who had received the least.

I showed that those who had received the most vaccinations had three times as many days off work, sometimes with very serious and disabling illnesses, as those who had received the least vaccinations.

When I presented my brief, I was given the last one and I was almost insulted by being told that it was a deplorable brief, very badly done and that it did not provide any proof. (If I had been in the presence of an honest jury, concerned about people's health, before this brief was presented, it would have helped me to make it from a more orthodox statistical work)!

So I was basically threatened not to get my diploma if I didn't take over this work completely. This is to tell you that the system is rotten from start to finish. What you have to understand is that the current medical world knows nothing about immunity.

What you need to know is that Jenner or Pasteur had no notion of the problems of immunity. It was only really at the time of AIDS, in the 1980s, that the extent and complexity of immunity began to be discovered.

What appeared then (around the 1990s) through work on stress, is that immunity involves a very complex axis with several levels of mutual interactions: psychological, neurological, hormonal and biological dimensions.

We cannot intervene on immunity without there being repercussions on one of these other levels. And as the vaccine community has no notion of these immunity data because they only have one criterion, it is very simple: it is the presence of antibodies or not... generally they study the tolerance of the vaccine.

What does this word mean? It means that during the trials, we're going to look at what happens around the vaccine in the next few days for molecules, proteins that are supposed to have an action of several years, 5 years, 10 years!

Is that honest? Does it make sense? What science is in there? There is nothing... and when I think that we are all trained on this model and that we are made to believe that everything is perfect and that it is the vaccines that have made diseases disappear... it is really enough to cry to pretend that it is a science!

You have to know that there is a tremendous manipulation about the disappearance of smallpox. The W.M.S. issued a document in 1980 when it decreed that smallpox had disappeared, in which it said:

"Eradication campaigns based entirely or mainly on mass vaccination were successful in a few countries but failed in most cases. »

The W.M.S. went on to say: "The abandonment of mass vaccination in favour of the so-called 'surveillance-dispersion' approach is of paramount importance. ...] It was possible in this way to completely stop transmission even when variola incidence was high and immunization rates low. »

The strategy of mass vaccination had therefore completely failed, and the simple strategy of quarantining infected people changed all that and succeeded in eradicating smallpox even in areas where this was not possible.

In India, for example, the W.M.S. carried out a mass vaccination in 1962 and in the years that followed, smallpox exploded! Mass vaccination was a total dead end.

In spite of this, the myth was forged for the whole medical world, including the WHO, that smallpox had disappeared thanks to vaccinations! This is the historical sleight of hand, and the whole history of vaccinations carries with it a deliberate lie, characteristic of today's medical environment.

The whole planet is threatened. Think about it: no philosophy, no religion has managed to get the agreement of all humans, yet all humanity has been vaccinated without any obstacles. How is this possible?

The worst victims of this whole system are children. When you think that from the first months of life, during the first year of life, the vaccination calendar provides for 18 vaccines (grouped together). This is indefensible!

When you think that a child's immune system needs to mature in 6 or 7 years, and the fundamental stage in the maturation of a child's immune system is childhood diseases.

Respect for the emergence of childhood illnesses is the place where children definitively expel energies, disturbing emotions and where their immune system is freed from the shackles of any past and at that moment it reaches the beginning of its maturity.

At that moment, the whole psychic, neurological, hormonal and biological space is freed and the child can develop to its full potential without obstacles. I am thinking of the health of the children and I ask for a minute of silence in honour of all these sufferings.

Our pharmacies are overflowing with pills that are useless and can even be fatal. In a 900-page book, medical professors Philippe Even and Bernard Debré sift through 4,000 medicines. The results are overwhelming: 50% of them are useless, 20% are risky and 5% are even "potentially very dangerous"!

But the taboo of vaccines is still there and it would probably have been far too much to realise that their criticisms could exactly extend to the practice of vaccination. All the more so as the vaccination approach has inaugurated the method of influence and manipulation in medical practice. Quite simply because vaccines inaugurated the first steps in the industrialisation of pharmacy combined with lobbying with the state.

Finally, and especially if they denounce the dangers of drugs, they seem to totally ignore the role of vaccines in the emergence and progression of chronic, autoimmune and degenerative diseases (which in fact becomes the blessed bread for all these new drugs they denounce).

In fact we are facing a situation of rupture, because medicine is at an impasse. The biochemical impasse. It is trying to find the molecules intervening at the DNA level to control the disturbances there. But this level is governed by a different type of electromagnetic influence.

DNA participates in two levels of reality: biochemical and electromagnetic. It is precisely very interesting to see this biophysical space appear in the structuring of living things at the cellular level. For forty years now, quantum physics has explored and determined the mechanisms of this interface at the DNA level (work by Popp, Gurwitsch, Driesch, Burr, Gariaev - see the site wavegenetic.ru). This biophysical space is governed by photon-based principles of light information.

Here we must underline a coherent convergence of our society. The internet revolution has shown how all human activities (information, transport, storage, sale...) are now monitored, governed, organised and controlled by electromagnetic devices. However, this situation is only a form of transposition of an active mechanism in complex biological spaces which use the same possibilities of instantaneous information transfer controlling and driving biochemical reactions (wave-particle complementarity).

A revolution that is struggling to fit into the understanding of the medical world, which is forty years behind these fundamental discoveries. Such a revolution would also be capable of rehabilitating medical practices that are discredited by official circles, such as acupuncture, homeopathy and chromatotherapy. But much more than that, it would make it possible to understand the reality of an interface between body and soul (also a taboo word in medicine) and to explain the mechanisms of NDEs (Near Death Experiences) and their consequences.

We can then better understand how this revolution in knowledge is struggling to emerge in the medical world, one of the most conservative (dare we say reactionary!) scientific spaces, which would thus be profoundly transformed to adapt to the complexity of living beings straddling physical and biochemical spaces.

The progress that is essential to finally open up the mystery of the living. A revolution and an indispensable development to open the reconciliation between man and his environment. This new way of seeing would give back to the human being a space of freedom able to better understand the mechanisms of energy and consciousness that run through him in total harmony with those of his environment.

A revolution even greater than the one that occurred in medicine with the anatomo-pathological revolution associated with all those great names in modern medicine Bichat, Laennec, (but also in science) and at the beginning of the industrial revolution. A revolution in phase with the social and political revolution of that time which inaugurated the industrial revolution of which we are living in the present impasse.

Interview with Mr Michel Georget, Associate of Biology

The journalist: *Michel Georget, you were a biology professor, you wrote the book: "Vaccinations, the undesirable truths", what led you to take a particular interest in the vaccination issue?*

Michel Georget: *As a young father, I was lucky enough to meet a family doctor who was not a fanatic about vaccinations and when I asked him the question: but then do we vaccinate or don't we vaccinate? He answered: yes, well, listen, I'm going to vaccinate your daughter, but you have to document yourself, you'll see that vaccinations are not a panacea and there are risks, you have to document yourself.*

So as I was a biologist, it was a good thing because I had access to university libraries and I quickly observed that the discourse that was written in the biology books used in secondary and high schools did not correspond exactly to reality.

Especially when one had access to Pasteur's documents, his laboratory notebooks, since Pasteur's family gave his laboratory notebooks to the national library. We realized at that point that the halo that we had given Pasteur was not entirely justified because there were of course experiments that were a bit rigged.

Later on, when I retired, as I had quite a few friends in the medical profession who knew I had documents on these subjects, they asked me to put it all in writing, they told me: you mustn't keep it to yourself, you have to write a book.

Journalist: *There is a lot of talk about the cervical cancer vaccine, what exactly is it?*

Michel Georget: *First of all, it's a vaccine that is not directly against cervical cancer but against cervical infection, which can, in the distant future, in some cases only lead to cervical cancer.*

So these are the latest vaccines on the market, and I'm all about information. The people who are offered, or even forced to be vaccinated must be informed about the risks of the disease of course, but also about the risks and effectiveness of the vaccinations.

In the case of the cervix, this is not done. This is real propaganda with inaccuracies and even real lies. Just one example: cervical cancer is often presented as the second most common female cancer after breast cancer, obviously this is frightening talk when in reality it is not true at all.

It's true worldwide because at least 80% of these cancers are in developing countries, but it's not true at all in developed countries and in Western Europe, depending on the country, cervical cancer is 14th or 15th among women's cancers, so it's a long way from breast cancer.

Among the lack of information concerning this vaccine is first of all the fact that, a little like hepatitis B, which has also been much talked about, HPV infection is spontaneously reversible in 90% of cases thanks to the immune system without any after-effects, and this is therefore also true for hepatitis B.

And when the infection leads to changes in the mucous membrane of the cervix, lesions can of course appear at different stages, but it should be noted that at all these stages, spontaneous regression can also occur.

These percentages are as follows: when the lesions are at the 1st stage there is 60% spontaneous regression, the remaining 40% can therefore evolve if we do not treat towards a 2nd stage where there 40% are still reversible, and at the 3rd stage 30% are still reversible. And in the end, if no precautions are taken, no treatment is envisaged, it can obviously, at that moment, evolve towards an invasive cervical cancer.

These are words that are much more reassuring than saying: this cancer is the second most common cancer in women after breast cancer. And what is also dramatic is that there is information that doesn't appear anywhere.

For example, I found on an official site of the Canadian Ministry of Health that, for vaccines and generally speaking, this is also true for this vaccine against papillomavirus, no research on reproductive toxicity is required for vaccinations.

But here we are dealing with vaccines that affect the genital sphere, and what is to be feared is that in a few years perhaps we will find ourselves with problems comparable to those caused by Distilbene, this drug, this synthetic hormone that was taken by women about thirty years ago during their pregnancy and which led to cancers for these women and especially to genital anomalies and cancers in the descendants.

The daughters of these mothers who were treated with Distilbene had great difficulty in having children and today we are talking about the next generation, the grandchildren whose daughters and even boys may present anomalies of the genital apparatus and even develop cancers.

This is therefore an example of the transmission of drug toxicity through the generations and it is not at all impossible that such toxicity could also be found in the vaccine against cervical cancer.

Speech by Françoise Joët (Alis association) at the Mutualité on 24 November 2009

Ladies and gentlemen, I speak here tonight on behalf of thousands of people who refuse to see their health and that of their children endangered by hazardous and systematic vaccine injections. Even if we do not hear them, thousands of voices are raised every day demanding the right to choose the best way to preserve the balance of health.

And if there is one area where the fundamental freedoms of the individual are flouted, it is that of vaccinations. For 200 years now, they have been practised, massively and blindly, and increasingly without the slightest scientific proof - I mean scientific proof of their effectiveness, usefulness and harmlessness. A paradox that has no equivalent in any other field.

Why is this? How did it come about? Well, since Jenner, and especially Pasteur, vaccination has become a dogma that has given rise to an unquestionable institution. This has allowed the gradual establishment of a state control over citizens in collusion with the pharmaceutical industry and the principals that are the major international health organisations and their accomplices who finance them.

Vaccination, therefore, is not a matter of health but of power and money. Nor is it a matter of knowledge, but of faith. In this context where power and commercial interests take precedence, it is not surprising that all kinds of excesses are possible: mass vaccinations with the hussar, especially in the Third World, the addition of more and more toxic products to vaccines for maximum profitability, a heavier vaccination schedule, no precautions before vaccination and no follow-up afterwards, no exhaustive information either from the public or from doctors, no vaccino-vigilance, no recognition of post-vaccination accidents, with very rare exceptions after a course of combat for the victim, make-up of data and propaganda with the complicity of the major media.

And finally: voting on vaccination obligations accompanied by sanctions, fines, prison sentences, suppression of parental rights, dismissals, blackmail in hiring, persecution and bans on doctors' practices.

This picture, which may seem unbelievable to you, is the true face of vaccinology. Behind the mask lies a sad reality that has put disease in the place of health and submission in the place of conscience. As a result, the consequences of a policy of false prevention through vaccination are very heavy, both in the medical field and in the field of ethics and law.

On the one hand, the health of populations throughout the world is deteriorating with the emergence of new diseases - more than 5,000 rare diseases are currently listed - or the resurgence of old diseases. All this is due to the pressure to select germs or to their mutation favoured by vaccinations.

On the other hand, we see the intrusion into our societies of new problems that we do not know how to solve and which generate colossal expenses. This is the case with autism, behavioural disorders and degenerative diseases that affect increasingly younger people.

From an ethical point of view, forced vaccinations are unquestionably an attack on physical integrity, even though they are defended by the Constitution and French law, as well as European law. Imposing vaccinations also leads to abuse of trust through the use of lies and fear. Especially when parents are led to believe that a baby absolutely needs a whole collection of vaccines before the age of 2, when his immune system cannot cope.

In addition, intolerable pressure is exerted on society in the name of vaccination coverage when the health is solely that of the individual, a principle reaffirmed in 1997 in the Doviedo Convention which states that the interest and good of the human being must prevail over the sole interest of society and science. All European states have signed it, and this is fundamental.

So what are we asking for? Well, first of all, that vaccination no longer escapes the law and that we stop violating the Constitution with direct or indirect vaccination obligations.

This presupposes, first of all, respect for democratic laws that guarantee the fundamental freedoms of the individual. Secondly, it presupposes respect for the code of medical ethics. And finally, thirdly, it presupposes respect for the precautionary principle and its corollary, the principle of prudence. When in doubt, one should abstain and not persist.

We would add that mass vaccinations, which have never solved anything and which are akin to a life-size experiment, must stop, thus endorsing the massacre of a certain number of innocent people.

Furthermore, the new scientific knowledge in biology, virology, immunology, etc. must be taken into account, and this must lead to a questioning of the practice of vaccination and its validity. Current scientific data integrate a vision of the microbial world that is totally opposed to that of pasteurism.

It goes without saying that, for all these reasons, it is high time to establish a rigorous assessment of the vaccination policy which must be carried out by specialists who are totally independent of the pharmaceutical and financial lobbies.

For years, the association I represent - Alis - has been suggesting to parliamentarians that they vote for a conscience clause to be granted to all citizens. Several bills have already been proposed but never examined due to a lack of political will.

I will conclude by saying that our societies will not survive if their citizens continue to suffer what they do not approve of and which degrades their health. That from now on, thanks to the Health Alliance, and it is our wish, a society of men and women will be built that knows how to regain their sovereignty and their freedom, the freedom of their bodies being an essential requirement.

One last sentence: it is the choice of life and not the choice of destruction that we must make, the only guarantee of the durability and good functioning of our democracies.

France has infected the entire planet

How sad to note that it is our country, France, that has infected all the countries of the world with this unnatural theory of vaccination, injecting the metastases of this veritable cancer of medicine into all the health systems of the planet.

Thus the United States has declared war on all opponents such as Barbara Loe Fisher, president of the National Vaccine Information Center, who has been fighting for 34 years to defend life and human rights. This is her historic speech to the Minneapolis Congress on Health Freedom in 2014. Thanks to Citizen Initiative for permission to reproduce it and the following speeches, all taken from NVIC.

"These little wonders are the most precious gifts that Life gives us. As soon as they are born, they never cease to amaze us. We feel we love them with all our heart and more than anything else. These little ones love and trust us like no one else ever will.

And... one day we realise that they have grown up, that they are making their own life and that they, in turn, are holding their own babies in their arms. This is the natural order of life.

But this natural order, many small children will never know it. Some are already dead, others will join the ranks of the handicapped, others will grow up and die in state institutions with adult bodies and baby brains. For these children, the natural order of things will have been changed forever by man-made vaccines that they were legally forced to receive.

Today, one of the most important topics of conversation concerns our freedom of choice: do we still have the freedom to choose how we will maintain our physical health, our mental health, our emotional health, our spiritual health? These questions ultimately lead us to examine complex scientific, philosophical, legal, economic and cultural policies.

What unites all those who enter the open debate on vaccination and health is the commitment to defend physical integrity, as well as the inalienable right to self-determination which has been globally recognised as a fundamental human right. Among the most debated health-related issues is the question of whether individuals can disagree with official health policies, as well as the right to exercise their freedom of thought, speech and conscience about vaccinations.

Vaccination is a medical act that has been promoted to a sacrosanct status by those who control the official medical system. Vaccination is proclaimed to be the most important scientific discovery and medical act in the history of medicine.

Using religious symbols and "crusading" rhetoric, proponents of vaccination describe it as a true Holy Grail. They claim that vaccines will eradicate all causes of disease and death on earth. And those who doubt it are nothing but foolish ignoramuses.

In the 1970s, Dr. R. Mendelsohn, Pediatrician, who described himself as a medical heretic, wanted to warn the people that science had become a religion and that vaccination had become his new sacrament.

In the 21st century, if you refuse to believe that vaccination is a civil and moral duty, and if you dare to question the safety of vaccines or claim the legal right to refuse one or more government-recommended vaccines, you run the risk of being labeled heretical, anti-scientific, a traitor threatening public health and, as such, you only deserve to be humiliated, silenced and punished for your protest.

Freedom of thought, speech and autonomy

"To find out who imposes his law on you, you simply have to find out who you are not allowed to criticise," said Voltaire, the great 18th century writer from the Age of Enlightenment. Voltaire was imprisoned several times in the Bastille because he wanted to defend freedom of thought and speech before the French Revolution.

There has never been a better time than now to challenge those who want to rule our health with an iron fist. We have the power, and everything we need.

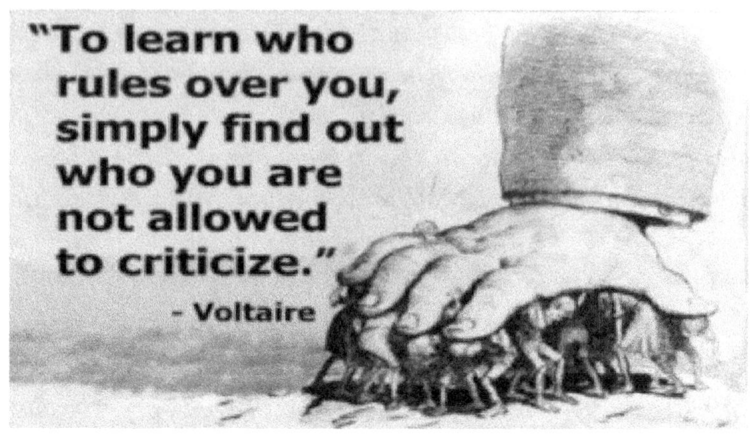

Information is power

In the 21st century, we have the necessary tools to enter a new age of Enlightenment in order to liberate the people and allow them to regain their freedom and health. The Internet allows us to bypass the bought media, dominated by industry and governments. Internet allows us, thanks to our computers, tablets, smart-phones, to communicate widely and publicly what has happened to our health, to our children's health after vaccinations.

We are connected to each other in ways we have never been connected before, **and it is high time to talk about vaccines, germs and the real causes of poor health.** It is high time to face our fears and stop believing that we and our children will get sick, will die if we do not believe and do not carry out the orders of those we have given the power to manage our health care system with an iron fist.

A free people has the power to reject the sole recourse to a single, often expensive, some say ineffective, medical model that has dominated health care affairs in the United States for nearly two centuries now. [...]

A free people can refuse to buy genetically modified food. A free people has the power to distance itself from doctors who threaten and punish patients who refuse to obey their orders to get annual flu shots, or to have their children receive the full recommended vaccination programme without them being able to ask questions or claim exemptions.

The most rational and compelling arguments in defence of health freedoms, such as immunization, are based on ethics, law, science and economics. The human right to free and informed consent to vaccination is the best example that should, without further delay, make Americans stand up for their inalienable right to autonomy and protection of their physical integrity.

At NVIC, we strongly encourage the Hippocratic principle of **"first do no harm".** At NVIC, we do not argue for or against vaccines. We support the legal and fundamental right to make informed and voluntary health decisions, such as choosing to get all the vaccines recommended by the government, some of them only, or no vaccines at all.

With NVIC, we are acting in an environment that is becoming more hostile every day and is created by the medical trade alliance, industry and government who want to pass laws that would force all Americans without exception to make all officially recommended vaccines or to undergo the sanctions provided for.

The people of California have stood up to defend exemptions from vaccination. **In 2012, many Californians traveled to Sacramento to protest a law** introduced by a pediatric congressman that would make it more difficult to obtain exemptions from immunization based on personal beliefs.

These citizens responded to our calls and marched in front of the Capitol buildings, sometimes accompanied by their children, sometimes waiting for hours to present their testimony to the crowd. Mums, dads, grandparents, nurses, doctors and chiropractic students followed one another in front of the microphones to present their testimonies, talk about the health damage suffered and sometimes death.

Californians inspired the citizens of Colorado to stand up in 2014.

The actions, letters, e-mails, testimonies, appeals launched by Californians in 2012 encouraged Colorado residents to follow this good example when the personal belief exemption was attacked in Colorado. This time, there were a sufficient number of Colorado legislators who bowed to the evidence.

All the efforts of the citizens paid off, as they were able to maintain the personal belief exemption (vaccination).

Albert Einstein risked arrest in Germany in the 1930s when he spoke out against censorship and persecution of minorities. It was then that he said: ***Never do anything against your conscience, even if the state asks you to.*** It takes a lot of strength to act independently. When the whole herd is running straight towards the cliff, the one running in the opposite direction can only look crazy.

Gandhi: ***Say what you think!***

Ghandi was often persecuted by the majority who ruled the country for challenging their authority. He used civil disobedience to demonstrate his political protest. He said: "Never apologise for being upright and correct, for being ahead of your time. If you are right and you are sure you are right, say clearly what you think. Even if you are the only one in the minority, the truth will always remain the truth. »

Sharing what you know to be the truth will give courage to others to make choices according to their conscience.

Vaccination is not a patriotic act

There is no more fundamental freedom and no more inalienable natural right than the freedom to think independently, and to follow one's conscience when it comes to choosing what might risk our life or that of one of our children. And that is why informed and voluntary consent in relation to a medical risk is a fundamental human right. Despite the propaganda spread by paid experts, getting vaccinated is by no means a patriotic act, and refusing a government-recommended vaccine is by no means a criminal act. It is simply a choice.

Although we are born equal, we are not all the same

Vaccination must depend on a choice because, although we are all born equal, with equal rights under the law, we are not all the same. Each of us is born with different genes, a unique miocrobiome influenced by epigenetics which influences the way we respond to the environment in which we live.

We do not all respond in the same way to infectious diseases and we do not all respond in the same way to pharmaceuticals such as vaccines. Public health laws that do not respect biodiversity and force everyone to be treated the same are dangerous and unethical.

My son had a severe reaction to the Diphtheria-Tetanus-Pertussis vaccine

When my son Chris started to suffer from convulsions, shock and inflammation of the brain within hours of his Diphtheria-Tetanus-Pertussis (acellular) vaccination, I understood for the first time what it meant to be a member of a minority. He was two and a half years old at the time.

The inflammation of the brain following the vaccine was followed by regression.

The inflammation of the brain, also known as encephalopathy that my son Chris suffered from after his DTPa vaccination was followed by a progressive deterioration of his physical, mental and emotional condition, not to mention chronic infections, recurrent diarrhoea, new allergies, lack of progress, loss of previous gains, inability to concentrate, and changes in personality and behaviour.

The risks of trusting without verification

What happened to my son, who was perfectly healthy in 1980, made me want to learn more and try to understand why doctors don't talk about vaccine risks and especially why a commercial product that can damage the brain and kill people could be made compulsory.

Why did I irrationally believe that vaccines were 100% safe and effective? Why did I put blind trust in the doctor instead of studying vaccination with the same zeal that I had shown when I researched nutrition, exposure to toxic products during pregnancy, childbirth with or without an epidural, breastfeeding or bottle-feeding?

A whole journey to find answers

Some of my questions have been answered during the two years of research I have been doing with medical historian Harris Coulter. I learned that the pertussis vaccine contains a dangerous toxin, an endotoxin, as well as aluminum and mercury that can make the blood-brain barrier permeable.

This research led to the publication in 1985 of our book: DPT: A Shot in theDark. Harris and I were the first to report an association between inflammation of the brain and dysfunctions that doctors call seizures, learning disabilities, attention deficit and autism. But it would take another 25 years of research and contact with politicians, doctors in industry and government to be able to answer the other questions that remain unanswered.

Every person knows someone...

In 1982, when I contacted parents who had children whose health had been damaged by the DTP vaccine, and when I founded the National Vaccine Information Center, the number of Americans who questioned the safety of vaccines was so small that a survey probably could not have shown anything.

Three decades later, national polls show that the majority of American parents admit that their number one health concern is vaccine safety.

The explanation for this is simply that every person knows at least one other person who was healthy, got vaccinated, and then never experienced good health again.

Militarisation of vaccination policy: fear has taken the place of trust

Mothers usually ask their doctors logical questions about vaccination. But when doctors sometimes react to these questions with irrational rage or an outright refusal to continue medical care when mothers refuse certain vaccinations, it becomes perfectly clear that something is wrong when doctors feel they have to promote and force the use of a pharmaceutical product.

The militarization of vaccination policy in the United States is eroding the trust that existed between patients and their doctors, and it is fear that has taken the place of this shattered trust. And then in the United States, we have gone from 23 doses of 7 vaccines to 69 doses of 16 vaccines. One of the reasons why people are asking more and more questions about vaccines is that there have been major changes in vaccine policy since 1982.

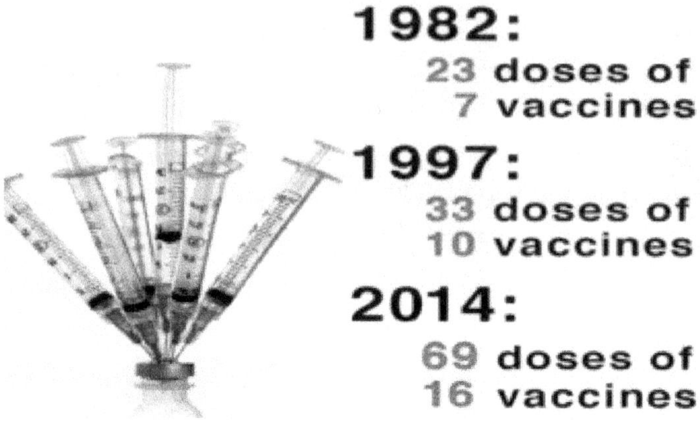

1982:
23 doses of
7 vaccines
1997:
33 doses of
10 vaccines
2014:
69 doses of
16 vaccines

Utilitarian justification transformed into law

It is important to note that at the beginning of the 20th century, in the case of Jacobsen V. Massachusetts, the Supreme Court clearly relied on utilitarian justifications in deciding that a minority of citizens who opposed vaccination should be forced to be vaccinated in the service of the majority. Today, utilitarian thinking has a more banal and pretty name. It is called the "greater good".

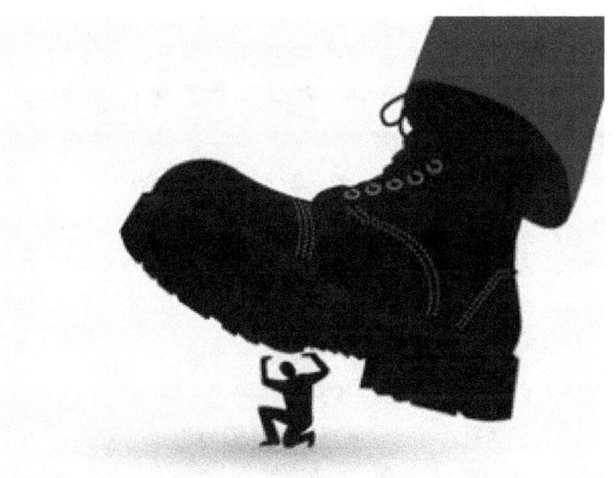

Militant utilitarianism puts minorities at risk

...] The Third Reich used utilitarian thinking as an excuse to demonise minorities deemed to be a threat to the welfare of the state. With the support of health officials, the very first minority that was considered to be in need of sacrifice were severely handicapped children, the chronically ill, the mentally retarded, in short the "useless eaters" as they were called.

The list of people who were labelled as posing a threat to health, economic stability or state security continued to grow to include minorities of people who were too old, too Jewish, too Catholic, too adamant in their opinions, or simply those who did not want to believe that what the state leaders were saying was true. This was the list of people who were stigmatised by the state, and who had to be demonised, isolated, feared, followed closely, isolated...

Utilitarianism is a discredited pseudo-ethics

Utilitarianism is a discredited pseudo-ethics that has been used to justify horrific human rights abuses, not only during the Third Reich, but also in relation to scientific experimentation on humans, the inhuman treatment of prisoners or political dissidents in many countries. This is why this principle should never be allowed to serve as a guide in any policy or in the creation of laws by any government.

While we cannot agree with the quality and quantity of scientific evidence used by governments to declare vaccines safe at the population level; while the state may have the power, it certainly does not have the moral authority to decree that a minority of individuals born with certain genes or biological susceptibilities must give up their own lives, without their consent, because the majority in power felt that this was what has been called "the greater good".

Our lives are defined by the choices we make

The road we take in this life is defined by the choices we make. If we are not free to make our choices, the road we take in life is no longer our own. The choices we make, it is true, can include risks to our bodies that house our minds. But these choices are among the deepest choices we can make in this life. That is why we must be free to make them.

Sicker than previous generations

Americans don't know that their children have to get more vaccinations than any country in the world requires. Children and young adults are sicker today than generations before them. We are witnessing epidemics of chronic diseases and many disabilities.

Vaccinated from the first day of life!

There is still so much that scientists don't know about the development and functioning of the immune system.

In 1991, the CDC decreed that all healthy infants born to healthy mothers should be vaccinated against hepatitis B within 12 hours of birth.

Hepatitis B is a blood-borne disease that is most prevalent among adults who use drugs intravenously or who have multiple sexual partners.

Furthermore, in the United States, hepatitis B has always been rare in infants and children. The recombinant hepatitis B vaccine is the first genetically modified vaccine that has been approved by health authorities in the United States. This vaccine was tested on only a few hundred infants born to hepatitis B-infected mothers before the CDC recommended that pediatricians give the vaccine to every healthy newborn born to healthy mothers. Pharmaceutical companies, health officials and doctors now allow themselves to manipulate the immune system of the developing fetus in the mother's womb.

It all started in 2006. CDC officials advised obstetricians to give pregnant women a flu shot every trimester.

In 2011, Diphtheria-Tetanus-Pertussis vaccine was added to the vaccination programme for every pregnant woman, although this vaccine has not been licensed for routine administration to pregnant women. - CDC officials are telling doctors that it is okay to give these vaccines to pregnant women every three months, no matter how short the time between pregnancies.

The purpose of this practice is to replace the passive immunity naturally acquired and transferred from mother to baby with the artificial immunity given by the vaccine. The FDA (Food & Drug Administration) classifies these four vaccines as category B or C drugs for pregnant women. This means that there are no adequate controlled studies that can prove that these vaccines are very safe for the development of the foetus or for the pregnant woman. It is again worrying to realise that once again "boilerplate" vaccines have overtaken real science.

In 2013, an Institute of Medicine once again recognised that there were huge gaps in vaccine science. It acknowledged that doctors cannot predict which children will suffer from the side effects of vaccines.

The Institute of Medicine also concluded that the vaccination programme recommended by the CDC has not been adequately and scientifically evaluated for safety. It specified: the key elements of the entire (vaccination) programme, the number, frequency, order, timing and age of the vaccines; these elements have not been examined during studies and research.

Is the children's immunization program safe?

Does the war on micro-organisms make our world safer or does it compromise the biological integrity of the human race? I don't think it is wise to fool Mother Nature, or to upset the balance of her wonderful plans.

On top of all these unanswered questions about vaccination and health, we are witnessing an unprecedented war against freedom of thought, freedom of expression, against the very autonomy of people here in America.

Senior doctors who create and sell patented and recommended vaccines are allowed to interfere in federal immunization policy. In addition, these people are applauded when they allow themselves to tell doctors and parents that a child can, without any problem, receive up to 10,000 vaccines at a time.

Universities receive money from pharmaceutical companies and the government to conduct clinical trials on vaccines, while self-proclaimed bioethics experts and professors call for the criminalization of those who refuse vaccines. So parents can be charged with murder if one of their unvaccinated children transmits an infectious disease to another person who dies from it! [...]

Paid ideologues and propagandists are busy orchestrating hate campaigns on the Internet to damage the reputation and destroy the careers of doctors, scientists, journalists, lawyers, celebrities and parents who question the safety of vaccines and call for vaccine freedom.

Pressure is being put on doctors and nurses who vaccinate to turn a blind eye to the fact that we are not all the same.

Everyone without exception must be a candidate for vaccination. Even people whose immunity is severely compromised are advised to get most vaccines. We vaccinate people with cancer and AIDS. Previous side effects of some vaccines are overlooked because they are not important. This is why people take the liberty of vaccinating again.

And...when something serious happens, we talk about coincidences. There is a collective denial that vaccines have nothing to do with a whole series of side effects. At whatever level, no one is responsible - the manufacturers, the sellers, those who authorise, recommend, make the different vaccines compulsory.

It is one thing for the government to make vaccinations available to the public, who will ultimately have the freedom to choose; it is a completely different thing to intimidate the people:

No vaccine? No school

No vaccine? No job

No vaccine? No medical care

No vaccine? No insurance

No vaccine? No visa

Is the day approaching when we will no longer be able to get a driver's license, fly, get tax breaks, rent a hotel, or shop if we can't provide proof that we have received all the doses of all the vaccines recommended by the government?

This situation is likely to happen if Americans don't decide to stand up today to take the matter to court, to appeal to the legislature, to trumpet information publicly so that we can finally put limits on the power of those who, with an iron fist, run the health care system. [...]

Science is not static, doctors are not infallible and we are not all the same. If the state is allowed to intimidate people into injecting biological products of known or unknown toxicity, then there will be no limits on the freedoms that the state will allow itself to take away in the name of the greater good.

However, the signs are there to show us that it is not too late to forge a new destiny where true health, freedom, personal life, the wisdom of nature, and our need to live in harmony with it, will finally have their rightful place. In the midst of the suffering and oppression we perceive all around us, we see a wonderful awakening of people who no longer want to be sick and powerless.

It is wonderful to be alive, to struggle, to be engaged and to witness this awakening of humanity that will sweep away an outdated and deadly paradigm so that a new and luminous consciousness can emerge. We will not stop, we have faith in the truth. Our mission continues. We do not want mandatory vaccinations in the United States!

Extracts from Barbara Loe Fisher's speech of December 1, 2015.

"2016 will be the 34th year that I fight for vaccine security and human rights. For more than 20 years I have warned that the day would come when vaccine extremists and profiteers would work to create laws that would force Americans to buy and receive government-mandated vaccines, as well as to punish those who would refuse.

Still, it was a shock to me that all this has already happened in California and that extremists are preparing to attack religious and conscience exemptions in other states next year.

...] I was raised with deep respect for the values and beliefs on which our Republic was founded, as well as respect for the natural rights and democratic principles outlined in the United States Constitution.

...] This year, when extremists and profiteers used the few cases of measles that occurred in Disney Land to attack freedom of speech, freedom of thought, freedom of religious belief, my heart was heavy. It was really painful to see that there was no longer any hesitation in demonising good people who had done nothing but criticise inadequately tested vaccines and inhumane all-purpose vaccine policies.

And when dozens of medical bills pushed by the pharmaceutical industry and the medical world were introduced in several states to eliminate exemptions on grounds of conscience or religious grounds, it took my breath away. Now we were going to be able to track down, discriminate, isolate and punish those who did not want to comply with government policy.

What were the people going to do? Would they bow down and cower before their oppressors or would they stand up for their basic rights and civil liberties?

...] Congress suggested that the Federal Health Agencies create commercial partnerships with the pharmaceutical industry. Politicians gave extremists and profiteers the money and power to do whatever they wanted, without taking legal responsibility for their actions, including

forcing citizens to pay for and receive dozens of injections of vaccines or being denied the right to schooling for children, access to medical care and employment.

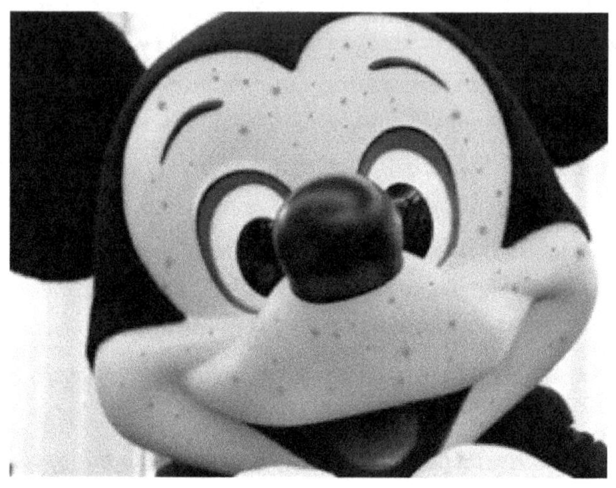

We are experiencing the greatest public health disaster in our country's history:

1 in 45 children (who have received a full range of vaccines) is autistic in America today; 1 in 6 children suffer from learning disabilities, 1 in 9 children suffer from asthma, 1 in 10 suffer from attention deficit hyperactivity disorder; 1 in 12 people suffer from depression; 1 in 400 people have become diabetic and millions more suffer from other forms of autoimmune diseases, brain disorders with chronic inflammation of the brain or body. So many children have inflamed brains or bodies, an inflammation maintained by an under-tested federal vaccine program.

These vaccines, which are injected into pregnant women, like the very first day of birth, artificially manipulate the immune response and induce inflammation that may never go away. It will take a lot of muscle, energy and money to keep our ship from sinking. Waking people up is the first step. Everyone must get involved and vote for men and women of integrity who can defend our freedoms. The second step is to stop voting for anyone who threatens our freedom.

Desperate situation for those who deny the risks of vaccines

These are indeed desperate times for those who continue to deny the risks of vaccines. We know this because we are witnessing so many acts of desperation by doctors determined to end the public debate on vaccination and health. Those who want to deny the risks of vaccines are working hard to restrict public access to information, cover up vaccine damage and deaths, and arrange to violate the fundamental right to free and informed consent.

No flu shots? No jobs!

2013 had barely begun when public health agencies and professional medical associations demanded that nurses and health care staff be fired if they refused to obey orders to get flu shots - there were no exceptions and no questions could be asked. It didn't matter that the vaccine was risky, ineffective and almost useless against the strains that are most prevalent this year in the US.

Bill to make the vaccine mandatory

This first step was followed by legislation supported by health authorities and medical professional associations funded by pharmas such as the American Academy of Pediatrics in the states of Texas, Oregon, Arizona and Vermont. Their goal was to eliminate or restrict exemptions from immunization to give more power to physicians to compel children and adults to undergo immunization - with no exceptions and no questions asked"

Institute of Medicine Report: Where can you find the real science of vaccination?

In mid-January, the Committee of the Institute of Medicine published a report that opened the eyes of some. The report acknowledged that only 37 scientific studies had examined the safety of the current US vaccination schedule for newborns and children under 6 years of age, which includes a total of 49 doses of 14 vaccines compared to the 23 doses of 7 vaccines recommended in 1983. Due to the lack of a sufficient number of good scientific studies, the Committee was unable to determine whether or not the number of doses and timing recommended by the government was or was not associated with the development of chronic health problems such as seizures, autoimmunity problems, allergies, learning disabilities, and autism in the first six years of life.

Prevalence of autism in the United States: 1 child in 50

In March, a report was published by the National Centre for Health Statistics. The report estimated that among children attending school in the United States, 1 in 50 children had been diagnosed with an Autism Spectrum Disorder (ASD). In 2004 it was 1 in 150 children, in 1992 1 in 500, and in 1986 1 in 2,000.

In April, which is Autism Awareness Month in the United States, there has been widespread pressure from doctors inside and outside government to reject any association between the sharp increase in the number of vaccines given to children over the past 30 years and the corresponding sharp increases in autism cases in children.

These doctors knew, but many parents today still don't know, that the public debate about vaccine-induced brain inflammation, chronic brain disorders and immune dysfunction, including autism, began 16 years before a study was published in The Lancet in 1998 that examined the possible association between the MMR (Measles, Mumps, Rubella) vaccine and autism.

The CDC does not confirm Dr. Offit's claim that 10,000 vaccines are safe for babies. (CDC: American Centers for Disease Control).

On Friday, April 1, a study conducted and funded by the CDC was published in the Journal of Pediatrics. The study stated that "increasing exposure to antibody-stimulating proteins and polysaccharides in vaccines is not associated with a risk of autism" and therefore vaccines do not cause autism. It was in fact a pathetic attempt to validate a Machiavellian hypothesis put forward in 2002 by vaccine developer Paul Offit, who claimed that a child could react without problem to the administration of 10,000 vaccines at the same time.

However, any science student with a basic understanding of health research methods, and who knows about the effects of vaccine ingredients and the difference between naturally acquired and vaccine-induced immunity, could easily understand that in the absence of an unvaccinated control group, the study would be fatally biased. In fact, this study did not prove anything at all about the possible relationship between the administration of several vaccinations in early childhood and the development of autism among genetically different children with or without increased biological susceptibility to adverse reactions to vaccination.

Paediatricians describe parents in social networks as "troublemakers".

On April 15, Pediatric News published the results of an online survey that presented a truism: in social networks, a person's knowledge, values and beliefs, as well as the opinions of friends and family, strongly influence decisions about vaccination. Parents who express doubts about the safety of vaccines and use alternative immunization schedules have been pejoratively labelled as "troublemakers".

Pediatricians who commented on the survey suggested that "troublemakers" parents did not base their decisions about vaccines on "rational logic" and "scientific evidence" because they were influenced by "troublemaker" friends and misleading information on non-conformist and "troublemaker" sites. Apparently, no account was taken of the fact that the so-called "troublemakers" parents could not be convinced by poor science and the empty rhetoric that advocates boilerplate vaccines.

Journalist and magazine attacked for questioning Gardasil's safety

Also in April, a veteran journalist and radio host was personally attacked by pediatricians and public health officials in Buffalo, New York, for daring to write an article questioning the safety of the Gardasil vaccine and urging parents to make informed choices about vaccines. Indignant doctors threatened to financially ruin the magazine that published the article and to withdraw all paid advertising if the article was not removed.

Offit attempts to demonize "troublemaker" parents

At the end of April, a CNN journalist quoted doctors who blamed the pertussis, measles and mumps epidemics on unvaccinated people in developed countries because they were spreading doubts about the safety of vaccines on the internet, thereby endangering the world's health. Dr Offit's reaction was not long in coming: "It's the upper middle class, the well-educated white parents who are turning their backs on vaccines. These people usually have higher education, hold management positions and are used to controlling everything," he said flatly.

Doctors who have gone into the blame and criticism game don't even agree among themselves that the "troublemakers" parents who question vaccines are just stupid and irrational people, or perhaps well-educated, wealthy, white people who would refuse to acknowledge the intellectual superiority and infallibility of those who hold the titles of doctor of medicine, doctor of science, regardless of the colour of their skin or the money they make.

Doctors Offit, Halsey, Plotkin, Omer, and others who deny the risks of vaccines are busy criticizing everyone except themselves over the sad statistics that show that 1 in 50 children in America develops a type of immune and cerebral dysfunction called autism, whereas previously, before the number of vaccines given to babies tripled, there was only 1 case in 2,000 children.

Regression to poor health after vaccination: a universal experience

What the doctors who indulge in denial refuse to accept is that today everyone knows someone who was in good health, who was vaccinated and who, afterwards, never felt well again. This regression to a state of ill health, this kind of universal experience of suffering and risk after the use of a pharmaceutical product has a long and well-documented history.

These risks and failures explain why the public debate on health and vaccinations will continue into the 21st century and must continue. This debate will continue until doctors (who are pushing children and adults, already more vaccinated and sicker than ever before), to receive more and more vaccines, will finally decide to come up with better explanations than: "it's the fault of bad genes", "today we have better diagnoses" or "it's all coincidence".

Vaccine manufacturers and doctors, who are effectively immune from liability, nevertheless have a strict ethical duty.

In the United States, vaccine manufacturers are immune from liability in the civil courts. Doctors who promote and administer vaccines are also immune from lawsuits in the event of vaccine complications.

Physicians who are immune from legal liability, however, have a greater ethical obligation to encourage their patients and the parents of minor children to learn as much as possible about the risks of vaccines. They also have a moral obligation to respect the decisions of patients and parents, even if they personally do not share the decision taken.

Freedom of thought, speech and conscience is constitutionally protected in the United States. Public confidence in the integrity of public health policy is destroyed when physicians fail to respect the right to informed consent in relation to medical risks and when they act as intimidators in place of compassionate healers whose primary goal is to do no harm in the first place.

Human beings have experienced two centuries of vaccine orthodoxy. This orthodoxy wants us to believe that vaccination is effective and safe, and that governments should make it compulsory. It all began with the insistence of doctors that all people should accept the smallpox vaccine. It exploded in the last century when the US government wanted every child to receive 69 doses of 16 vaccines.

This vaccination orthodoxy had to be applied to every disease, every vaccine and every person regardless of their needs or sensitivities.

Today, everyone knows people who were healthy, who were vaccinated, and then never recovered. And when, for a person we love, the risks of vaccination are 100%, the most logical attitude to take is to become more informed so that such a thing can never happen again.

Paediatricians: guardians of vaccination knowledge

When I was young, the place where you could acquire knowledge for free was the city's public library. I took advantage of it to read history, art, biology, philosophy and literature. Then, in the 1960s, I joined the group of women who enrolled in university. I was then able to access a university library to learn even more.

When I became pregnant in the late 1970s, one of the first things I did was go to the library to read books on pregnancy, childbirth, nutrition so that I could give my baby the best start in life. But strangely none of these books contained information about the risks of vaccination. The paediatricians who were the guardians of vaccine knowledge did not share information about vaccine reactions with mothers. However, they wanted to make them understand that they were following the Hippocratic principle of "first do no harm".

It was the lack of knowledge that explained why I could not identify the classic symptoms of brain inflammation that occurred in my child within hours of the fourth injection of the diphtheria-tetanus-pertussis vaccine.

1982: Parental Protests about Vaccine Safety

Unhappy that I did not have the knowledge that would have saved my child, I joined the group of parents whose children's health had been damaged by vaccines, and finally launched a new American movement for vaccine safety and informed consent.

It was 16 years before a British doctor wrote an article about the MMR vaccine and autism; 26 years before a Hollywood star explained how her son developed autism after vaccination; and 34 years before $3.3 billion in compensation was awarded to vaccine victims who had suffered *brain and immune system disorders (National Childhood Vaccine Injury Act).*

Knowledge is power

It was the third President of the United States, Thomas Jefferson, who said: "Knowledge is power; knowledge is security, and knowledge is happiness. "Jefferson has always been a famous defender of education and free thought. He was the one who guaranteed freedom of religion, freedom of expression, freedom of the press. He considered these freedoms to be the most important rights enshrined in the First Amendment to the U.S. Constitution.

Yet today in America, when we take the initiative to educate ourselves about vaccination and infectious diseases, we are publicly labelled "ignorant" and "selfish" if the knowledge we have just acquired leads us to disagree with the orthodoxy of vaccination. Knowledge is power, and as a 19th century poet put it so well: "doubt grows with knowledge". It is not surprising, then, that doctors who are the guardians of knowledge about the risks, secrets and myths surrounding vaccination feel threatened in the 21st century by those who have decided to have free access to the "online medical library" and who have the audacity to engage in uncensored conversations about vaccines.

Educated parents reject vaccine orthodoxy

A growing number of studies show that educated middle-class parents who have taken the trouble to find out about the vaccine have come to reject its orthodoxy. In response, those who control and profit from the mass immunization system do not hesitate, according to orthodoxy, to use conventional propaganda techniques to persuade lawmakers to make immunization mandatory for all Americans or to subject them to penalties that trample on civil and human rights.

Last year at this time, we witnessed an unprecedented media campaign, bordering on hysteria, to castigate a few cases of measles at Disneyland. All this cinema to justify the removal of personal belief exemptions from California's education and child care system. Parents who opposed mandatory immunization were demonized. There was even talk of imprisoning them. There has also been online censorship in the public debate about vaccine risks and failures. Even doctors who questioned the safety of vaccines had their licences revoked.

This year has already begun to humiliate all those who reject the orthodoxy of vaccination. On New Year's Eve, the editorial of a Colorado newspaper did not hesitate to describe as "weird," "crazy," and "irresponsible" all those who do not want to bow down and conform to the government's dictates. It was even said that a law had to be passed to force these people to comply.

Two days later, a national business magazine targeted a Jewish family doctor practicing holistic medicine for criticizing the safety of vaccines and opposing a ban on children of Jewish families from attending summer camp if they had not received every dose of vaccine on the federal immunization schedule. He was accused of being "a threat to public health"! At that time, it was suggested that doctors who, like him, were critical of the orthodox vaccination schedule should have their licenses revoked.

Vaccine deaths and injuries do not discriminate in any way

Vaccine deaths and injuries do not discriminate on the basis of race or class, except when people are kept in the dark, economically dependent and unable to make informed choices. As more and more women in America, regardless of race or social class, are graduating from university, they will surely learn more about the risks of immunization when they become mothers.

This is one of the reasons why we are witnessing an acceleration of government and industry efforts to eliminate the right to free and informed consent with respect to vaccine risk in America.

Those who bow to vaccine orthodoxy are entitled to their beliefs, but it would be wrong to give them the legal right to persecute and punish fellow citizens who refuse to comply. Whatever it is called, tyranny will always be tyranny.

Standing up for civil liberties and human rights

As long as we still have freedom of speech, of the press, of thought, of conscience and of religion in America, we must exercise it at every opportunity.

If we all stand up to fight and defend the rights that have, unfortunately, already been lost, we have every chance of not losing more tomorrow.

Knowledge is the antidote to vaccine orthodoxy because knowledge is power.

Subscribe to the NVIC Newsletter and The Vaccine Reaction newspaper to keep yourself as well informed as possible. Learn how to identify and report vaccine reactions. Take the time to read the leaflets of the vaccine manufacturer(s)...

Take advantage of the year 2016 to regain your power by learning more about vaccine science, vaccine policy and the law. Don't hesitate to become a teacher and pass on your knowledge to your family, friends, and community leaders. You don't know how many lives you may be able to save. It's your health, your family, your freedom to choose! »

Large demonstration in Sacramento on 9 June 2015 and hearings in the California Parliament against Bill SB277, which would make vaccinations compulsory and remove exemptions.

"This bill (SB277) has nothing to do with measles or whooping cough," says Barbara Loe Fisher, President of the National Vaccine Information Center. Essentially, it wants to take away the power of fathers and mothers to make choices about medical issues that put their young children at risk, and put that power back in the hands of doctors. In this way, a blanket vaccination policy will be implemented without anyone taking any responsibility for any damage."

Crucial testimony from one of the victims of the mysteriously concealed vaccines during a hearing at the Sacramento Parliament

My name is Joshua Coleman and this is my son Otto (6 years old). When he was born Otto was in perfect health. At every visit to the paediatrician, Otto was given a series of vaccinations. He received all the vaccinations as per the official schedule. When Otto was 17 months old, he received four vaccines that contained six different valencies. At that time, he walked, ran, and "climbed" just like little boys his age.

One morning when I went into his room, shortly after he had received his 6 vaccinations, I was scared to death because he couldn't stand up. We immediately took him to the emergency room. Over the next few days Otto had to endure a painful lumbar puncture, a brain scan and an MRI. It was discovered that he was suffering from an autoimmune reaction called transverse myelitis. The doctors explained to my wife and I that his immune system had become confused and started attacking his own spinal cord, causing severe damage.

We asked why all this had happened. The doctor told us it was most likely a reaction to a vaccine, or a virus. The latter was immediately rejected because Otto had shown no signs of illness. Then the doctor slammed the door shut, ending any discussion that might have helped us understand how our son who was healthy and could walk had suddenly become paralyzed.

No further investigation was made to determine what caused our little one who was walking and running to suddenly find himself in a wheelchair for the rest of his life. Later we took our little boy to John Hopkins Hospital for further tests. There the doctors looked at all the possible reasons for our son's paralysis. All possible reasons except for vaccinations.

It didn't make sense and it still doesn't make sense today when every doctor who had examined Otto at four different hospitals had mentioned that the vaccinations our son had received in the vicinity of his paralysis might be the most likely culprit.

As parents we are reliving the moments before our son's paralysis to try to see more clearly in this situation that went wrong. We think we are revisiting the fact that we had absolutely no opportunity to give informed consent to what was done to our 17 month old son in that doctor's office.

The paediatrician did not ask us about our family history. Our pediatrician did not ask us if Otto, my wife or I were allergic to any of the ingredients in the vaccines our son was going to receive. Nor did he review the leaflets with us, contraindications, possible side effects, warning signs to allow us to be on the lookout for any signs that would require immediate medical intervention as is done with any other kind of prescribed medication, except vaccines.

Not only did he not go through all of this with us, but he did not even show it to us so that we could see it! He also failed to mention that not a single vaccine has ever been tested according to the golden scientific standard, that of a double-blind, placebo-controlled study (neutral or saline solution).

Instead, vaccines are tested against other vaccines, combinations of vaccines, adjuvants or ingredients that may themselves cause harm. To add to the shock and horror, the combination of multiple vaccines that are given at one time has never been studied, despite the fact that they are given in random order, in multiple combinations day after day to millions of children!

Not a single doctor thought to contact the FDA, CDC, CHPH or HHS after the damage our son suffered after the vaccination. Not a single doctor has made any reports to the VAERS (Vaccine Adverse Event Reporting System) as required by the National Vaccine Damage Act of 1986.

Of all the doctors we consulted, not a single one told us about the VAERS, their legal obligation to send a report or suggested that we write a report ourselves. Blood samples were never sent to experts for examination. The lot numbers of the multiple vaccines that Otto received were never reported to possibly detect "hot lots" to make sure that what had happened to our son didn't happen to other children.

Let's realize how things would have taken a whole new turn if Otto had contracted mad cow disease from a hamburger he ate: calls would have been made immediately, reports would have been filed immediately, an investigation would have been launched immediately. Warnings would have been issued, the media would have been alerted. When it comes to vaccine damage or death after vaccines, none of this happens. As a result, Otto is now stuck in a wheelchair.

To add insult to injury, not a single doctor had the decency and compassion to tell us about the Vaccine Injury Compensation Program (VICP). By the time we heard about it from other parents, it was legally too late to file a complaint for our son Otto...the short 3 year statute of limitations had expired.

So we had to survive on the income from a single treatment because of the constant care that Otto's paralysis required. The entire burden of providing for the family's needs, as well as the huge hospital bills, rested entirely on the shoulders of one person. The 75 cent surcharge levied on each vaccine, the only insurance policy for parents against vaccine damage, was paid in pure loss. We were in fact denied the possibility of filing a complaint.

Tragically, Otto's case has done absolutely nothing. The suffering he is now enduring, his permanent disability, nothing will be done to prevent these misfortunes from affecting other children. Your child or grandson could very well be next.

Please try to imagine my extreme frustration, the frustration of many other parents present at this hearing today when we hear people in this room cavalierly claiming the lie that "vaccines are safe". Please ask yourselves, how could vaccines be completely safe as touted by Senators Pan and Allen, when at the same time the United States Supreme Court and Congress has declared them "unavoidably unsafe", in other words, inherently dangerous?

It is not just government regulators or vaccine manufacturers who recognise that vaccines can harm and even kill. This is now common knowledge because of the increasing number of victims. That's why more and more Californians opposed to the new bill are attending the hearings. They outnumber supporters by 15 to 1.

So the vaccine damage is very real and not as rare as we are led to believe. And it is parents who want to be able to choose the risks they want or don't want to take for their children. If vaccine damage is rare, as the bill's proponents say, one complication per million doses, there should be no more than 39 people (vaccine victims) before the 39 million-strong state parliament today. Can I please ask for a show of hands? ... How many of you have had a child who has been vaccinated or have been vaccinated themselves? It seems to me to be well over 39 in a single room!

I hope you will now understand why my wife and I can never again, in good conscience, allow Otto to receive a single vaccine. The same goes for his younger brother. As there has been no investigation, we have no idea which vaccine ingredient or combination of ingredients has or have caused the paralysis. We are determined not to blindly sacrifice our children on the altar of vaccines any longer. These vaccines we know are dangerous and poorly studied. We would have preferred to take the risk that our children would get the (natural) disease rather than receive these multiple vaccine injections. We know enough about this to be able to say that we no longer want them.

If this bill were to pass, Otto would risk not being able to go to school. It is unbelievable that he is not entitled to a medical exemption. If Bill SB277 passes, Otto will no longer be able to attend public school. And I repeat... my wife and I will never again allow him to receive even one vaccine.

Otto has paid the ultimate price and he will never be the same again. As a token of thanks, his most basic right to normal schooling has been taken away. Home schooling does not suit us financially or practically.

Are you, Senators, going to vote to take away his right to go to school?

»

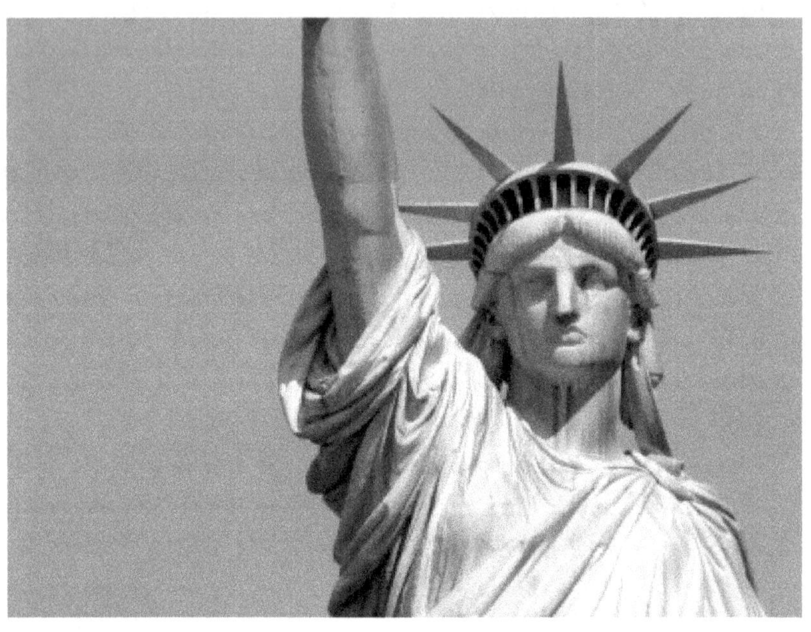

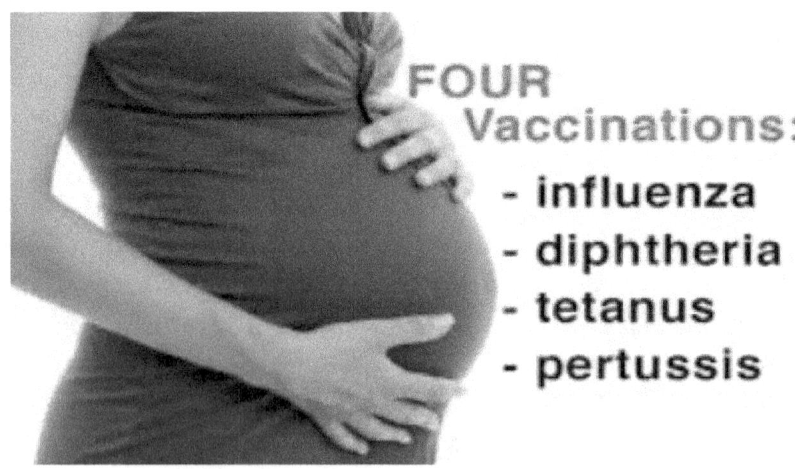

The disastrous effects of vaccinations

Professor Louis-Claude Vincent declared and demonstrated, through bioelectronics, that "Nobody escapes the consequences of vaccinations, in the short, medium or long term".

Doctor Guylaine Lanctôt, in her book, La Maffia Médicale, draws up a small and terrifying list of the complications caused by vaccinations:

In the short term:

- the disease itself or its atypical forms: pertussis cough, polio-like paralysis, etc.

- allergies

- urticaria (giant)

- eczema

- exanthemas (redness)

- asthma

- malaise

- painful inflammation

- local reactions

- swollen lymph nodes

- anaphylactic shock that can lead to death

- fever

- kidney damage

- purpura

- oedema (swelling)

- rheumatism

- gastrointestinal disorders

- sudden infant death syndrome 1 to 3 weeks after the vaccine

- all acute diseases of the nervous system :

- severe to mild encephalitis

- panencephalitis (measles vaccine)

- meningitis

- irreversible neurological damage

- Guillain-Barré syndrome
- cerebral palsy
- major brain damage
- Vaccinal infarction in the 30-40 age group
- hepatitis B
- fetal alteration or death

In the medium term :
- neurological disorders:
- autism
- brain damage :
- convulsions
- hyperactive child
- incessant crying
- appetite disorders (anorexia/bulimia)
- damage to cranial nerves (blind/deaf/mute/dyslexic)
- hypotonia
- delayed development
- cerebral palsy
- mental problems :
- mental retardation
- behavioural disorders
- personality disorders
- intellectual disorders
- learning disabilities
- hypersexuality
- emotional instability
- juvenile delinquency
- sociopathic personality
- criminal behaviour
- childhood leukaemia
- repeated infections
- numerous allergies

In the long term :
SAFE EFFECTS :
- imbalance of our organism
(individual ecology)
- weakening of our immune system
- (natural defence)
- upheavals within our cells: permanent alteration of chromosomes
(DNA), malformations, etc.
- Introduction of foreign proteins transmissible to the genetic code
of a species
(new training courses)
CONSEQUENCES :
- multiple sclerosis
- leukaemia
- cancers
- AIDS
- congenital malformations
- infertility
- chronic fatigue syndrome
- epilepsy
- Parkinson's disease
- cardio-vascular diseases
- multiple allergies
- degenerative diseases :
- Alzheimer's disease
- lupus
- arthritis
- re-emergence of old drug-resistant diseases
- emergence of new unknown diseases :
- congenital malformations
- hereditary genetic defects
- mutations in the human species

- Threat of extinction of the human race

Don't miss out!

Visit the website below and you can sign up to receive emails whenever ANDRÉ HUAN publishes a new book. There's no charge and no obligation.

https://books2read.com/r/B-A-FLBN-JGULB

BOOKS 2 READ

Connecting independent readers to independent writers.

www.ingramcontent.com/pod-product-compliance
Lightning Source LLC
Chambersburg PA
CBHW050524160726
48003CB00001B/453